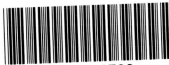

Management of Colorectal Cancers in Older People

Demetris Papamichael • Riccardo A. Audisio
Editors

Riccardo A. Audisio
Series Editor

Management of Colorectal Cancers in Older People

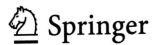 Springer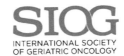
INTERNATIONAL SOCIETY
OF GERIATRIC ONCOLOGY

Editors
Demetris Papamichael, MB, BS, FRCP
Bank of Cyprus Oncology Centre
Nicosia
Cyprus

Riccardo A. Audisio, MD, FRCS
University of Liverpool
St Helens Teaching Hospital
St Helens
UK

Series Editor
Riccardo A. Audisio, MD, FRCS
University of Liverpool
St Helens Teaching Hospital
St Helens
UK

ISBN 978-0-85729-983-3   ISBN 978-0-85729-984-0   (eBook)
DOI 10.1007/978-0-85729-984-0
Springer London Heidelberg New York Dordrecht

Library of Congress Control Number: 2013933444

Springer is part of Springer Science+Business Media (www.springer.com)

Contents

Contributors

Riccardo A. Audisio M.D., FRCS Department of Surgery, St. Helens and Knowsley Teaching Hospitals, St Helens, Merseyside, UK

Leïla Bengrine-Lefevre, M.D. Oncology Department, Saint Antoine Hospital, Paris, France

Luigi Bonanni, M.D. HPB Unit, North Manchester General Hospital, Pennine Acute Trust, Manchester, UK

Elisabeth Carola, M.D. Oncologie Médicale, GHPSO, Senlis, France

Priya Das, MBBS Royal Berkshire NHS Foundation Trust, Reading, UK

Aimery de Gramont, M.D. Department of Medical Oncology, GERCOR, Paris, France

Department of Medical Oncology, Hopital Saint-Antoine, Paris, France

Nicola de' Liguori Carino, M.D. HPB Unit, North Manchester General Hospital, Pennine Acute Trust, Manchester, UK

Eduardo Diaz-Rubio, Ph.D. Oncology Department, HC San Carlos, Madrid, Spain

Gunnar Folprecht, Ph.D. Medical Department I/University Cancer Center, University Hospital Carl Gustav Carus, Dresden, Germany

Bengt Glimelius, M.D., Ph.D. Department of Radiology, Oncology and Radiation Science, Uppsala University, Uppsala, Sweden

Rob Glynne-Jones, FRCP, FRCR Mount Vernon Cancer Centre, Middlesex, UK

Margot A. Gosney, M.D., FRCP Elderly Care Medicine, University of Reading/Royal Berkshire NHS Foundation Trust, Reading, Berkshire, UK

Siri Rostoft Kristjansson, M.D., Ph.D. Department of Internal Medicine, Diakonhjemmet Hospital, Diakonveien, Oslo, Norway

Valery E.P.P. Lemmens, Ph.D. Department of Research, Comprehensive Cancer Centre South, Eindhoven, The Netherlands

Department of Public Health, Erasmus University Medical Centre, Rotterdam, The Netherlands

Gerrit-Jan Liefers, M.D., Ph.D. Department of Surgery, Leiden University Medical Center, Leiden, Netherlands

May Mabro, M.D. Oncologie, Hopital Foch, Suresnes, France

Aranzazu Manzano, M.D. Oncology Department, HC San Carlos, Madrid, Spain

Kannon Nathan, MRCP, FRCR, B.Sc. Clinical Oncology, Mount Vernon Cancer Centre, Middlesex, UK

Harm J.T. Rutten, M.D., Ph.D., FRCS (London) Colorectal Surgery, Catharina Hospital Eindhoven, Eindhoven, Noord Brabant, The Netherlands

Zenia Saridaki, M.D., Ph.D. Laboratory of Tumor Cell Biology, Medical School, University of Crete, Heraklion, Crete, Greece

Javier Sastre, Ph.D. Gastrointestinal Unit, Oncology Department, HC San Carlos, Madrid, Spain

John Souglakos, M.D., Ph.D. Medical Oncology, Medical School University of Crete, Heraklion, Crete, Greece

Andrew P. Zbar, M.D. (Lond), MBBS, FRCS (ED), FRCS (Gen), FRACS, FCCS, FSICCR (Hon) Surgery and Transplantation, Chaim Sheba Medical Center, Tel Hashomer, Ramat Gan, Tel Aviv, Israel

Jon Zugazagoitia, M.D. Oncology Department, HC San Carlos, Madrid, Spain

Chapter 1
The Epidemiology of Colorectal Cancer in Older Patients

Valery E.P.P. Lemmens

Abstract One of the most commonly diagnosed types of cancer at an older age is colorectal cancer (CRC). The median age at which CRC is diagnosed nowadays is 69 years. Due to the aging of the population and the fact that individuals between 80–89 years exhibit the highest risk of being diagnosed with CRC, the median age at diagnosis will further increase in the near future. An important feature of elderly cancer patients is the fact that they often present with comorbidity. Among patients with CRC, the prevalence of comorbidity has been increasing over the last decades. Among patients aged 80–89 years old the prevalence of comorbidity increased from almost 60% in 1995–1998 to 80% in 2007–2010. Also tumor location shows a relation with age. With the exception of appendiceal tumours, older age is related to a more proximal tumor location within the large bowel. Older patients are less often diagnosed with node positive disease, as wel as synchronous distant metastases. Also socio-economic status of patients with CRC shows a strong relation with age. Of patients younger than 55 years, 18% of the patients is of a low socio-economic status, while this amounts to 42% among patients aged 80 or above. Five-year elative survival of patients with CRC decreases by age, from 66% for patients younger than 45 years old, to 55% for patients older than 75 years. Survival has been improving recently also for elderly patients. This, together with the increase in incidence, will lead to an increased prevalence of elderly with CRC. This development will increasingly ask for investments in clinicalresearch and infrastructure with a special attention for the elderly patient with CRC.

Keywords Epidemiology • Colorectal cancer • Older patients • Elderly • Survival • Comorbidities

V.E.P.P. Lemmens, Ph.D.
Department of Research, Comprehensive Cancer Centre South,
Zernikestraat 29, P.O. Box 231, Eindhoven 2600 AE, The Netherlands

Department of Public Health, Erasmus University Medical Centre,
Rotterdam, The Netherlands
e-mail: v.lemmens@ikz.nl

D. Papamichael, R.A. Audisio (eds.), *Management of Colorectal Cancers in Older People*,
DOI 10.1007/978-0-85729-984-0_1, © Springer-Verlag London 2013

Introduction

In the forthcoming decennia the number of elderly will rise in the Western society, not only because the first postwar baby boomers have meanwhile reached the age of 65 but also because life expectancy continues to rise. The average life expectancy at birth in Europe is estimated to reach 89 years for women and 84.5 years for men in 2050 [1]. Since the risk of most of types of malignancies increases by age, the number of elderly patients with cancer consequently will increase as well. However, not only demographics are responsible but also lifestyle-related factors such as the increased prevalence of smoking among women and the changing patterns in sun exposure contribute to the expected increase in the number of patients with cancer. Last but not least, the ongoing drop in mortality of "competing" diseases such as cardiovascular diseases may as well partly be responsible for a further increase in the number of elderly patients who develop cancer. One of the most common types of cancer at older age is colorectal cancer. Between 65 and 85 years of age, it is the most common cancer together with lung and prostate cancer, while among individuals over the age of 85, colorectal cancer is most frequent together with skin and breast cancer [2]. Of all male patients with colon cancer, 91 % is over the age of 55, while 30 % is between 75 and 84 years old, and 7 % is 85 years or older at time of diagnosis. Among women even 13 % is aged 85 or older. Only non-melanoma cancer and cancer of the stomach and bladder are characterized by a higher proportion of patients aged 85 or more at time of diagnosis.

Incidence

In Fig. 1.1 the age-specific incidence of colorectal cancer is depicted per 100.000 inhabitants of the same age group, separately for males and females [2]. As an example specific for the Western population, the figures from the Netherlands in 2010 are used. The age-specific incidence is higher among males than among females, at all ages. Although the median age at which colorectal cancer nowadays is diagnosed is about 69 years, in Fig. 1.1 it can be seen that the highest risk of being diagnosed with colorectal cancer is between 80 and 84 years for males and between 85 and 89 years for females. This means that with an aging population – hence growing proportions of people aged 80–89 years – the median age at which colorectal cancer is diagnosed will shift toward an even higher age in the near future.

In the longstanding Eindhoven Cancer Registry in the Netherlands [3], trends over a longer period of time can be studied. When comparing the proportions of certain age groups over time with respect to age at diagnosis of colorectal cancer, it can be noted that the proportion of patients diagnosed below the age of 55 was 17 % in the period 1981–1985, which dropped to 10 % in 2005–2010. On the other hand, the proportion of patients diagnosed aged 75–79 increased from 14 to 17 % between 1981 and 1985 and 2005–2010, the proportion aged 80–84 increased from 9 to 12 %, and the proportion over 85 years of age increased from 5 to 8 %. This means

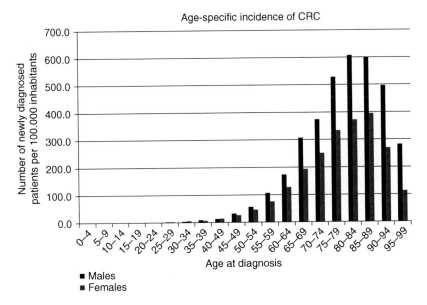

Fig. 1.1   Age-specific incidence of CRC (*Source*: Eindhoven Cancer Registry [4])

that the total proportion of patients older than 75 has increased from 28 % in the beginning of the 1980s to 37 % in most recent years.

Gender

The male–female ratio is showing a U-curve when compared between the respective age groups. Among patients younger than 55 years, 45 % of the patients is female (source: Eindhoven Cancer Registry). This drops to 40 % at the age of 65–69 years, but then steadily increases up to 48 % females among patients aged 75–79, 56 % among patients aged 80–84, and above the age of 85 even 65 % is female. Although the risk of colorectal cancer within the older age groups remains higher among men as we learned from Fig. 1.1, women at older age outnumber men, thanks to their higher life expectancy. This U-shaped male–female ratio remained rather constant within the last three decades.

Comorbidity

An important feature of older cancer patients is the fact that they are more likely to present with comorbidity. In Fig. 1.2, the prevalence of various types of comorbidity at the time of diagnosis among patients with colorectal cancer is presented by age (source: Eindhoven Cancer Registry). Hypertension, cardiac disease, and previous

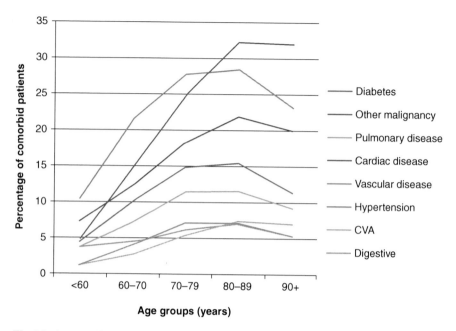

Fig. 1.2 Age-specific prevalence of comorbidity among patients with CRC, according to comorbid condition (*Source*: Eindhoven Cancer Registry [4])

malignancies (excluding basal cell carcinoma of the skin) are the most frequent comorbid diseases. A large increase for all types of comorbidity with increasing age can be noted, the age-related increase being largest for cardiac disease. The prevalence of comorbidity keeps increasing up to the patient category aged 80–89 years, thereafter the prevalence slightly decreases, which may in part be explained by some underreporting or by a selection of fitter patients who lived long enough to develop cancer. Also striking is the high proportion of patients with previous malignancies – up to 22 % of patients aged 80–89 already had a previous diagnosis of cancer. From Fig. 1.3 it becomes clear that the prevalence of comorbidity is increasing over time, across all age groups. Of patients aged 70–79, 57 % suffered from comorbidity in 1995–1998, which rose to 72 % in 2007–2010. For patients aged 80–89, almost 80 % had comorbidity in the most recent period. Also after adjustment for age, the increase in prevalence of comorbidity among patients with colorectal cancer remained significant. Looking at the various types of comorbidity, there was, for example, no increase in COPD, but there were large increases on the other hand for diet- and physical activity-related comorbidity such as hypertension, cardiac disease, and diabetes. The prevalence of diabetes, for example, rose from 9 to 18 % among patients with colon cancer. In view of the effects of comorbid diseases such as diabetes on treatment and outcome, it is of high importance to address this issue in research and policy in terms of both prevention and management of colorectal cancer.

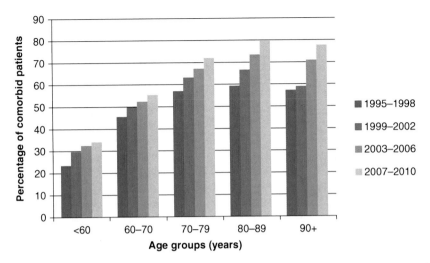

Fig. 1.3 Age-specific prevalence of comorbidity among patients with CRC, according to period of diagnosis (*Source*: Eindhoven Cancer Registry [4])

Anatomical Subsite

The distribution of tumors within the colorectum shows a strong relation with age. With respect to tumors located in the appendix, there is a clear preponderance for younger patients below the age of 55: 38 % of all patients who are diagnosed with an appendiceal tumor – which is a relatively uncommon tumor – is younger than 55 years (source: Eindhoven Cancer Registry). Two percent of all patients with colorectal cancer at this age has an appendiceal tumor, compared with 0.2 % of patients over the age of 85.

Nine percent of patients younger than 55 has a tumor located in the coecum, which becomes a more frequent tumor location with increasing age: of patients older than 85, 17 % has a coecum tumor. The same pattern can be observed in the colon ascendens, where 5 % of younger patients has their tumor located, compared to 12 % of the oldest patients. More distal, the pattern starts to change; in the colonic sigmoid, there is a U-shaped relation with age: somewhat less common in the youngest or oldest patients, but most common for patients 65–75 years old. Among patients younger than 55 years, 38 % has a tumor located in the rectum, while among patients over the age of 85, 24 % has rectal cancer. In general, with the exception of appendiceal tumors, older age is related to a more proximal tumor location. Remarkably, this relation is strengthening over time: for example, the proportion of patients under 55 years with a rectal tumor has increased over time, while in 1981–1985, 28 % of young patients was diagnosed with rectal cancer, this has now increased to 42 %. When choosing screening or diagnostic tools, this may be of importance, for example, sigmoidoscopy is more likely to miss tumors among older patients.

Stage at Diagnosis

Postoperative T stage is related to age to a certain degree: of patients who underwent resection younger than 55 years old, 9 % is diagnosed with pT1, while for patients aged 85 years or older, this is 7 % (source: Eindhoven Cancer Registry). This proportion drops from 19 to 15 % for pT2 and increases from 54 to 61 % for pT3. Interestingly the proportion of pT4 does not change with age: it comprises about 9 % at all ages. Also pTx remains constant over the age categories, at about 3 %. Concerning pN stage, the proportion with pN0 disease increases by age from 42 % among patients younger than 55–50 % among patients aged 80 or older. In this respect, it is of importance that the number of lymph nodes evaluated by the pathologist decreases by age. Finally, the proportion of patients with a positive M stage (including patients not operated on) decreases by age: from 25 % among patients younger than 55–13 % among patients aged 85 or older. This goes together with an age-related increase in the proportion with an unknown M stage. Probably, diagnostic procedures are used more sparingly among patients with a more limited life expectancy due to age and/or comorbidity.

Socioeconomic Status

There is a strong relation between socioeconomic status (SES) and age at diagnosis of colorectal cancer. Of patients diagnosed below the age of 55, 18 % is of low SES, while this amounts up to 42 % of patients aged 85 or older (source: Eindhoven Cancer Registry). Of the older group of patients, not surprisingly, a large proportion does not live independent anymore; 6 % of patients aged 75–79, 12 % of patients aged 80–84, and 23 % of patients over the age of 85 is residing in a nursing home or is otherwise institutionalized at time of colorectal cancer diagnosis.

Survival

The relative survival of patients diagnosed with colorectal cancer is decreasing by age; however, the age-related decrease is not dramatically high. One-year relative survival of patients with colon cancer is 86 % for patients younger than 45 years, 82 % for patients aged 45–54 years, 82 % for 55–64 years, 79 % for 65–74 years, and 69 % for patients older than 75 years [2]. The 5-year relative survival rates of the corresponding age groups are, respectively, 66, 60, 60, 59, and 55 %. For patients with rectal cancer, 1-year relative survival rates are 91 % for patients younger than 45 years, 89 % for patients aged 45–54 years, 88 % for 55–64 years, 84 % for 65–74 years, and 73 % for patients older than 75 years. The figures for 5-year survival of rectal cancer are 66, 65, 64, 62, and 52 % for the different age groups, respectively. In the last three decades, survival of rectal cancer has improved more than survival of colon cancer, thanks to positive developments in the treatment of rectal cancer, which will be addressed in other chapters in this book. Although several studies did not show improved survival rates for elderly with colorectal cancer, more recent studies do show a survival improvement also for the elderly, albeit smaller than among younger patients. Also elderly patients therefore seem to benefit from the developments in management of colorectal cancer.

Prevalence

The prevalence of colorectal cancer (meaning the sum of all patients with a colorectal cancer alive at a certain moment after diagnosis) is increasing due to the rise in incidence and the improved survival. This means that the weight that these patients put on the health system in terms of follow-up or treatment-related morbidity is growing. Within only 5 years, the 10-years prevalence (the number of patients alive who have had a diagnosis of colorectal cancer in the past 10 years) has risen in the Netherlands with almost 10,000 patients: from 50,417 patients in 2007 to 60,155 patients in 2011 [2]. This means a 20 % increase within only 5 years. This development is not expected to slow down in the forthcoming years; projections estimate a further increase in prevalence to over 90,000 patients in 2020 (so doubled within 14 years), a situation which is representative for Western Europe [4].

Conclusion

The number of elderly patients with colorectal cancer will continue in the forthcoming years. It is and will remain one of the most frequent cancers at high age. The median age at diagnosis will increase as well, which will go together with a higher prevalence of comorbidity. Besides this age-related increase in comorbidity, comorbidity itself is becoming more and more prevalent among patients with colorectal cancer probably related to lifestyle. Thanks to improvements in survival, recently also for elderly patients with colorectal cancer, the prevalence of cancer has been increasing. All of these developments will increasingly ask for investments in clinical research and infrastructure with a special attention for the elderly patient with colorectal cancer.

References

1. EUROSTAT. Available from http://epp.eurostat.ec.europa.eu. Accessed on June 1, 2012.
2. The Netherlands Cancer Registry. Available from http://www.cijfersoverkanker.nl. Accessed on June 1, 2012.
3. Eindhoven Cancer Registry. Comprehensive Cancer Centre South. Available from www.ikz.nl. Accessed on June 1, 2012.
4. Dutch Cancer Society. Cancer in the Netherlands until 2020. Trends and prognoses. Amsterdam; 2011.

Chapter 2
Genetic Alterations in Colorectal Cancer in Older Patients

Zenia Saridaki and John Souglakos

Abstract Colorectal cancer is typically associated with advanced age, with an estimated median age at onset which reaches 70 years of age in the western population. Limited data are available regarding the differences in genetic and epigenetic alterations in colonic carcinogenesis between younger and older patients. Some studies suggest that mutation status in critical genes, such as *KRAS*, *BRAF*, or *PIK3CA/PTEN*, is different, depending of the age at diagnosis of colorectal cancer. These data provide the evidence that distinct genetic mechanisms are implicated in the somatic development of colorectal cancer in younger and older patients.

Keywords Ageing • Genetic alteration • Colon cancer • Elderly patients

Introduction

The genetic underpinnings of CRC are especially well studied [52], and a multistep model for the carcinogenetic process in the colon epithelium, from normal mucosa to invasive cancer, has been proposed more than 20 years ago [17], as presented in Fig. 2.1.

This model implicates chromosomal aberrations, a phenomenon termed CIN for chromosomal instability and is associated with common somatic mutations, more frequently in the *APC*, *TP53*, and *KRAS* genes, followed in frequency by *PIK3CA* mutations [53] (Fig. 2.1). This model implicates the activation of the Wnt pathway,

Z. Saridaki, M.D., Ph.D.
Laboratory of Tumor Cell Biology, Medical School, University of Crete,
Heraklion, Crete 71110, Greece

J. Souglakos, M.D., Ph.D. (✉)
Medical Oncology, Medical School, University of Crete,
Heraklion, Crete, P.O. 1352, Voutes 71110, Greece
e-mail: johnsugl@gmail.com, j.souglakos@med.uoc.gr

D. Papamichael, R.A. Audisio (eds.), *Management of Colorectal Cancers in Older People*,
DOI 10.1007/978-0-85729-984-0_2, © Springer-Verlag London 2013

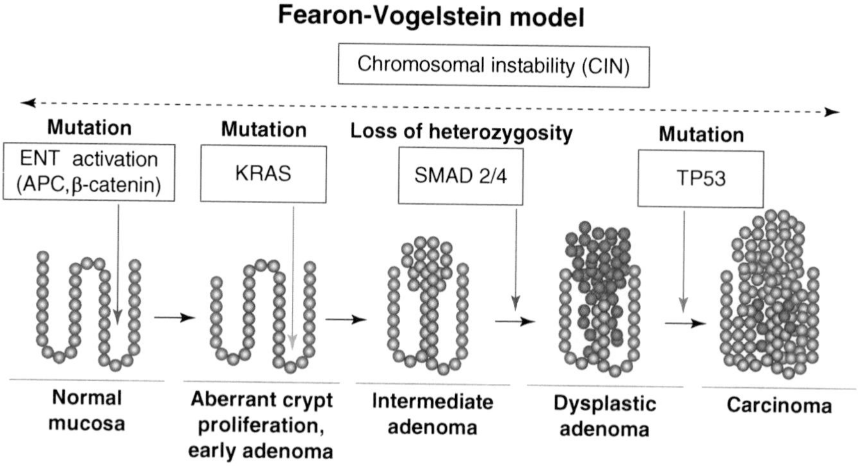

Fearon-Vogelstein model

| Chromosomal instability (CIN) |

| Mutation | Mutation | Loss of heterozygosity | Mutation |
| ENT activation (APC, β-catenin) | KRAS | SMAD 2/4 | TP53 |

| Normal mucosa | Aberrant crypt proliferation, early adenoma | Intermediate adenoma | Dysplastic adenoma | Carcinoma |

Fig. 2.1 The multistep process of carcinogenesis in the colonic epithelium with the corresponding genetic alteration in each step

through either inactivated mutations in the *APC* (more frequent) or *AXIN* genes or activated mutations of *beta-Catenin*. As a result, the aberrant proliferation of the cell in the crypt increases the level of genetic instability. The activated mutations in the *KRAS* gene lead to the formation of early adenomas. The subsequent loss of the tumor growth factor-beta (TGF-b) control on differentiation, through the loss of SMAD 2/4, leads to progression to advanced-dysplastic adenomas. Finally, the loss of the control to the genomic stability due to inactivated mutations in TP53 gene allows the formation of invasive cancers. For more than two decades, this model was considered as the only way for the initiation and progression of neoplasia in the colonic mucosa.

Subsequently, landmark experiments suggested that not all CRC present CIN. A subgroup of sporadic CRC, up to 15 %, is attributed to microsatellite instability (MSI) due to inappropriate mismatch repair (MMR) system [19]. This simplified approach suggests two paths to colon cancer, with all cases having some measurable degree of genetic instability, either CIN or MSI. The picture became more complex when it was reported that some colon cancers seemed to have neither MSI nor CIN [9]. Moreover, epigenetic changes marked by DNA methylation were increasingly described as a common event in colon cancers, and a specific pathway of intense DNA hypermethylation was identified, the CpG island methylator phenotype (CIMP) [28]. More recently, other epigenetic alterations such as histones modification and chromatin remodeling have also been described in subsets of CRC.

The potential clinical implications of multiple pathways leading to colon cancer are obvious and may change our approaches in all aspects, from prevention to screening to therapy. From a prevention standpoint, if the different colon cancers arise from different cells, it is likely that familial predisposition and carcinogenic exposures affect each pathway differently. Such heterogeneity in the disease initiation and natural history may explain the difficulties in reproducing some associations between exposures, lifestyle, and genetic polymorphisms on colon cancer risk. By extension then, interventions to prevent colon cancer may have a preferential effect on one disease type but not on others.

The major effect of the multiple pathways to colon cancer model relates to therapy. Despite decades of research, there continues to be uniformity in thinking of and in treating colon cancer. The different colon cancers have vastly different prognoses, ranging from favorable (MSI, BRAF unmutated) to very poor (CIMP, no MSI). Until now, with the exception of *KRAS* mutations as predictor marker of resistance to anti-EGFR monoclonal antibodies [1, 31], this knowledge in the biology of the disease has limited application in the daily clinical practice. In addition, there is no current model (including the classic "Vogelgram") that fit every patient with CRC. Finally, there are limited data regarding the differences in genetic alterations in colonic carcinogenesis between younger and older patients. These data are discussed in the next pages of the present chapter.

Human Ageing: Genetics and Biodemography

What is actually ageing and what causes it? Regardless of how much we have achieved in the ageing field, this is still a mystery. Self-evidently we can say that ageing is caused by macromolecular damage, since with age, homeostasis declines and damage accumulates. It is only relatively recently that we have discovered that ageing, like so many other biological processes, is regulated by transcriptions factors and signaling pathways. Although initial research was restricted to short-lived organisms such as worms and flies, nevertheless, it soon became evident that the findings applied to mammals as well. Astonishingly, mutational changes found to slow ageing, at the same time, postponed age-related disease, giving a whole new meaning to the field by presenting ageing as a potential therapeutic target [34]. In parallel to genes and environment, another factor which may affect ageing is chance [26].

One of the first discoveries conserved from yeast to primates was that dietary restriction extends lifespan by reducing the cellular damage accumulation rate through nutrient metabolism. But it soon became clear that dietary restriction attacks ageing by an acute and rapid decrease in the mortality rate [38]. We know now that this is accomplished through nutrient-sensing pathways involving the insulin/insulin-like growth factor (IGF-1) [3], the kinase target of rapamycin (TOR) [30], the AMP kinase [21], and the sitruins [36]. Other conditions that can increase lifespan are chemosensory and thermosensory signals, heat and oxidative stress, low ambient temperature, signals from the reproductive system, and reduction in translation and respiration rates [34].

Insulin/Insulin-Like Growth Factor (IGF-1)

This is the first and most well-studied pathway regarding its connection with ageing in animals, which, in addition, has been found to be evolutionary conserved [32]. Inhibiting insulin/IGF-1 signaling changes lifespan through changes (up- or downregulation) in gene expression of several transcription factors like the FOXO transcription factor, DAF-16, and the heat-shock transcription factor HSF-1 and SKN-1 [34]. In addition, the insulin/IGF-1 pathway senses nutrients and thus is a good candidate for mediating the longevity response to dietary restriction [33]. In worms [27], flies [11], and mice [3], dietary restriction extends lifespan through inhibition of the insulin/IGF-1 pathway, and in mice, a combination of mutations and dietary restriction can nearly double lifespan [5]. Completely knocking out the insulin/IGF-1 and PI3K pathways causes worms to live ten times longer than normal [4]. Furthermore, dietary restriction may inhibit cancer by downregulating insulin/IGF-1 signaling [29].

But can an insulin/IGF-1 activity perturbation increase lifespan in humans as well? Possibly yes. FOXO3A cohorts are located throughout the world, and variants of FOXO3A and AKT have been linked with longevity in several of them. Furthermore, in the German cohort, FOXO3A variants are found to be more frequent in centenarians than in 90-year-olds [40]. FOXO1 gene variants, as well, have been linked to longevity in American and Chinese cohorts [35]. In mammals, insulin levels rise in response to glucose, and this rise might shorten lifespan. In humans, conditions that inhibit insulin receptor signaling could actually promote longevity if the dietary glycaemic index was reduced [34]. Dietary restriction and nutrient sensors perturbation inhibit tumor formation as well, and mutations which increase lifespan during evolution probably also delay cancer, as cancer incidence correlates tightly with physiological ageing in different species [32].

Kinase Target of Rapamycin (TOR)

Inhibition of the TOR pathway increases lifespan in many species, and at least in *C. elegans*, it seems to activate a pathway which is distinct from the insulin/IGF-1 one, as it extends lifespan independently of DAF-16/FOXO [30]. TOR inhibition increases resistance to environmental stress consistent with a physiological shift toward tissue maintenance [34].

AMP Kinase

AMP kinase is an energy and nutrient sensor that represses anabolic and activates catabolic pathways when the cell's AMP/ATP ratio rises. In *Caenorhabditis elegans* again, AMP kinase overexpression has been shown to extend lifespan [2, 32]. In a way it mingles with the insulin/IGF-1 pathway since it can also extend lifespan in response to dietary restriction acting directly on DAF-16/FOXO [21].

Sitruins

Sitruins are NAD⁺-dependent protein deacetylases whose overexpression has been shown to extend lifespan in yeast, worms, and flies, but how exactly this is achieved is not clear yet [32]. In *C. elegans* though, sitruin overexpression seems to act by activating DAF-16/FOXO again.

Telomeres

Telomeres have been acknowledged as candidates for ageing determinants because they shorten with age. Their mode of action though is distinct from whatever is discussed above. Mice that are engineered to have longer telomeres live longer possibly because they are genetically modified to resist cancer. Telomere lengthening probably increases lifespan by preventing stem cell loss and certainly not by shifting the animal into a protective physiological state [48].

Telomere length (TL) is also associated with high cancer incidence. Recently, the results of a study where TL's differences between younger and older ($\geq$70 years of age) colorectal cancer (CRC) patients were assessed and correlated with survival [14]. The relationship between telomere repeat copy number and single gene copy number (T/S ratio) of peripheral lymphocytes DNA evaluated with qPCR was used as a surrogate value for relative TL. A borderline significant difference in TL (mean TL 0.981 versus 0.925 respectively; $p=0.067$) was observed when patients under and over 70 years of age were compared. When the assessment was repeated using four age groups (50–60, 60–70, 70–80, >80), a statistically significant difference in TL between the youngest and the oldest age groups was demonstrated (mean TL 1.022 versus 0.874, respectively; $p=0.02$) with evidence of shorter TL with advanced age. A marginal relationship was detected between overall survival (OS) and age (p-value$=0.066$) with older patients exhibiting slightly poorer survival [hazard ratio (HR) of 1.03, 95 % confidence interval (CI) 0.998–1.065], and no correlation was noted between relative TL and OS in the univariate and multivariable analysis. The authors concluded that their results validate the ability of a qPCR-based assay to differentiate between younger and older CRC patients with the use of TL, and this methodology is being used with the scope to evaluate the relationship of TL to treatment tolerance in elderly CRC patients [14].

Prospects for Human Interventions

Until recently the idea of lifespan extension was not a science project. Now we know that longevity can occur without debilitating trade-offs, and in long-lived mutants, many age-related diseases are delayed. The US Federal Drug Administration does not recognize ageing as a condition to be treated, as an indication; thus, for the time being, drugs affecting ageing will be approved only if at the same time they affect disease. Rapamycin, a TOR inhibitor, which is approved for human use for immune suppression has shown to extend the lifespan of mice even when administered late in life [23]. Drugs that are being developed to target age-related diseases, such as IGF-1 pathway inhibitors for cancer, may achieve extension of youth and life as well, but we do not know yet their potential or their side effects. It seems reasonable that drugs mimicking the effects of genetic mutations which extend lifespan might extend lifespan as well.

The Postponement of Human Senescence and Mortality

Senescence results from a cumulative imbalance between damage and repair. Progress in increasing repair (via medical intervention) and reducing damage (via public health preventing disease's strategies) are the two fundamental causes for health improvement [50].

Human senescence itself, as it was first documented back in 1994, has been delayed by a decade. This observation, as expected, has profound implications not only for individuals but also for society and economy. Mortality at advanced ages is being postponed because people are reaching old age in better health, not as a result of revolutionary advances in slowing the ageing process but as a result of ongoing and successful measures for improving health [50]. In countries with high life expectancies, the majority of children born since 2000 will arrive and celebrate their 100th birthday in the twenty-second century [10]. Although genetic factors have a modest role in determining the life longevity of individuals, nevertheless, the progress in postponing senescence is entirely due to medical revolution and public-health efforts, due to better education, rising living standards, healthier nutrition, and lifestyles. Since 1840 life expectancy has been increasing by more than 2 years per decade, and no imminent limit to further increases exist [39]. In addition it seems that weakness and frailness is being postponed as well. Prosperity and medicine are the two major factors contributing to postponement of senescence and debility. We cannot actively distinguish which is the most important because in many ways they interact with each other. Healthier populations are more productive and prosperous; prosperity allows access to better treatment, higher education, and more research [50].

In 1994, from a Swedish mortality data analysis, the first conclusive documentation that death is being delayed emerged. In the same year, two subsequent studies confirmed this finding in other countries as well. Since then, research is showing that postponement is continuing, and as a result of that, a remarkable increase in the numbers of centenarians is produced. From Aristotle's distinction between premature and senescent death, the widely accepted view was that the only cause of death at an advanced age is indeed old age and that nothing can be done about it. Thus, each species was thought to have a characteristic maximum upper limit of lifespan, which could never be overcome [50]. These notions, though, were recently contradicted [8, 12]. Mortality for humans seems to level off after the age of 110. Exceptionally long-lived people reach advanced age because they have a better state of health.

The search to discover genes related to major longevity has had little success, summarized to the modest effect of the two variants of the apolipoprotein E gene (APOE) [16, 20]. The theory of evolution as far as ageing is concerned supports that senescence is inevitable for all multicellular species [22]. Biodemography, though, has shown that this theory should be expanded in order to permit greater variations. Research in the laboratory and in the field confirms that for certain species and for certain periods of adult life mortality can decline with age. Furthermore, genetic, environmental, and dietary changes can substantially alter survival [22, 50].

In contrast with death, health is a difficult parameter to measure, and it is often unreliably documented. The prevalence of disease and morbid disorders among the elderly has increased over time, and part of this rise is due to earlier diagnosis of disease, like cancer and heart conditions [10, 50]. Most kinds of morbidity and disability, such as heart disease and dementia, lead to higher death rates. To achieve life expectancies of more than 100 years of age, novel knowledge will be needed. Genetic research will contribute to a deeper understanding of the mechanisms underlying senescence. Advances in research will potentially lead to prevention and more successful treatment of cardiovascular diseases and cancer [45]. Dietary restriction and other nongenetic interventions might also lead to strategies for delaying human ageing [38]. Although death reduction from any disease will not immediately and radically increase life expectancy, advances against many diseases acting synergistically will, especially because comorbidity is so common among the elderly. In this sense, geriatrics is becoming an attractive and important specialty, and research on ageing is now an engaging, proactive science with considerable funding from the authorities. Nothing in evolution can be understood except under the light of demography (and vice versa) because evolution is driven (and drives)by the dynamics of fertility, mortality, and migration of nonhuman species and humans as well [50]. Although the policy makers recognize that the world's population is ageing, they do not seem to realize that reform and change in the social, economic, and health-care system should be implemented in a faster pace. The twentieth century was the century of the redistribution of wealth, but the twenty-first will most likely be a century of the redistribution of work toward greater ages [51].

Mutational Profile of the CRC Genes in Relation to Age

CRC is typically detected in older people and has a median age at onset which reaches 70 years of age. Approximately 5 % of all CRC cases are diagnosed in patients younger than 50 years of age, and this early onset usually indicates an increased likelihood for genetic predisposition [6]. Nevertheless, the vast majority of these cases are ultimately regarded as sporadic, since no known genetic predisposition is found [37, 54].

The RAS-RAF-MEK-ERK-MAP kinase pathway mediates cellular responses to growth signals constituting an essential component of intracellular signaling from activated cell-surface receptors to transcription factors in the nucleus [41]. Some of the above-mentioned genes are critical molecular markers in CRC carcinogenesis and have already been incorporated in the treatment of CRC patients. Indeed, the knowledge of a primary tumor's *KRAS* mutational status is mandatory for the treatment of metastatic disease, since it is a predictor of resistance to monoclonal antibodies of the epidermal growth factor receptor (anti-EGFR moAbs) [7, 15, 24, 47, 49]. In addition, *BRAF* V600E mutation identifies a subgroup (less than 10 %) of patients with an exceptionally unfavorable prognosis [13, 46]; conversely, the presence of a defective tumoral DNA mismatch repair (dMMR) system seems to be a favorable prognostic factor, although these patients seem to fair worse with standard adjuvant chemotherapy [18, 25, 42, 43]. Furthermore, PTEN (phosphatase and tensin homolog) protein expression, and specifically its loss, seems to be associated in a number of studies with resistance to anti-EGFR MoAbs treatment [44].

In a study by Berg et al. [6], 181 CRC patients were included and divided into three age groups, younger than 50, 51–70, and older than 70 years old. Among the CRC patients, stratified by microsatellite instability status, DNA sequence changes were identified in *KRAS* (32 %), *BRAF* (16 %), *PIK3CA* (4 %), *PTEN* (14 %), and *TP53* (51 %). In the oldest patient group, MSI and *BRAF* mutations were statistically significantly correlated ($p < 0.001$), but no such correlation was found in the <50 age group. *KRAS* and *BRAF* mutation frequencies increased with patient age, both when comparing age groups and when age was considered as a continuous variable. In patients younger than 50 years old, *PIK3CA* mutations were not observed, and *TP53* mutations were more frequent than in the older age groups, implying that *PIK3CA* mutations are important for tumorigenesis among the elderly. No difference between the age groups was observed regarding *PTEN* mutations and aberrations.

Genome complexity, assessed as copy number aberrations, was highest in tumors from the youngest patients (<50 years old) group than from the >70 years old group. Contrary, the tumors from elderly patients had the highest gene mutation index, even though this group included fewer advanced stages. One could speculate that among the young patients, there are carriers with genetic predisposition.

A comparable number of tumors from young (<50 years) and old patients (>70 years) were quadruple negative for the four predictive gene markers (*KRAS-BRAF-PIK3CA-PTEN*); however, 16 % of young versus only 1 % of the old patients had tumor mutations in *PTEN/PIK3CA* exclusively. This implies that mutation testing for prediction of anti-EGFR treatment response may be restricted to *KRAS* and *BRAF* in elderly (>70 years) patients. Finally, *KRAS* mutant patients among the young age group were found to have significantly shorter survival than *KRAS* wt ones ($p = 0.02$).

In conclusion, in the study by Berg et al. [6], it was documented that the mutation status of the above-mentioned critical gene set varies depending on age at diagnosis and provides evidence of differences in the somatic development of CRC tumors in young and elderly patients. Nonhereditary CRC tumors in young patients have less gene mutations but more copy number aberrations across the genome, suggesting that some young patients may have an increase risk for cancer caused by alterations in genes involved in maintaining correct chromosome segregation. Distinct genetic differences found in tumors from young and elderly patients, whose clinical and pathological variables are comparable, indicate that young patients have a different genetic risk profile for CRC development than older patients.

Conclusion

The genetic alterations and subsequent molecular modification responsible for the initiation and progression of neoplasia in the colonic epithelium are the same between younger and older patients. The limited available data in the field support that colon cancer in elderly patients is associated with higher gene mutation index but less copy number aberration in comparison with tumors from younger patients. In addition, the incidence of *BRAF* mutations is higher in older patients.

References

1. Amado RG, Wolf M, Peeters M, Van CE, Siena S, Freeman DJ, Juan T, Sikorski R, Suggs S, Radinsky R, Patterson SD, Chang DD. Wild-type KRAS is required for panitumumab efficacy in patients with metastatic colorectal cancer. J Clin Oncol. 2008;26:1626–34.
2. Apfeld J, O'Connor G, McDonagh T, DiStefano PS, Curtis R. The AMP-activated protein kinase AAK-2 links energy levels and insulin-like signals to lifespan in C. elegans. Genes Dev. 2004;18:3004–9.
3. Arum O, Bonkowski MS, Rocha JS, Bartke A. The growth hormone receptor gene-disrupted mouse fails to respond to an intermittent fasting diet. Aging Cell. 2009;8:756–60.
4. Ayyadevara S, Tazearslan C, Bharill P, Alla R, Siegel E, Shmookler Reis RJ. Caenorhabditis elegans PI3K mutants reveal novel genes underlying exceptional stress resistance and lifespan. Aging Cell. 2009;8:706–25.
5. Bartke A. Insulin and aging. Cell Cycle. 2008;7:3338–43.
6. Berg M, Danielsen SA, Ahlquist T, Merok MA, Agesen TH, Vatn MH, Mala T, Sjo OH, Bakka A, Moberg I, Fetveit T, Mathisen O, Husby A, Sandvik O, Nesbakken A, Thiis-Evensen E, Lothe RA. DNA sequence profiles of the colorectal cancer critical gene set KRAS-BRAF-PIK3CA-PTEN-TP53 related to age at disease onset. PLoS One. 2010;5:e13978.
7. Bokemeyer C, Bondarenko I, Makhson A, Hartmann JT, Aparicio J, de BF, Donea S, Ludwig H, Schuch G, Stroh C, Loos AH, Zubel A, Koralewski P. Fluorouracil, leucovorin, and oxali-platin with and without cetuximab in the first-line treatment of metastatic colorectal cancer. J Clin Oncol. 2008;27(5):663–71.
8. Carey JR, Liedo P, Orozco D, Vaupel JW. Slowing of mortality rates at older ages in large medfly cohorts. Science. 1992;258:457–61.
9. Cheng YW, Pincas H, Bacolod MD, Schemmann G, Giardina SF, Huang J, Barral S, Idrees K, Khan SA, Zeng Z, Rosenberg S, Notterman DA, Ott J, Paty P, Barany F. CpG island methylator phenotype associates with low-degree chromosomal abnormalities in colorectal cancer. Clin Cancer Res. 2008;14:6005–13.
10. Christensen K, Doblhammer G, Rau R, Vaupel JW. Ageing populations: the challenges ahead. Lancet. 2009;374:1196–208.
11. Clancy DJ, Gems D, Hafen E, Leevers SJ, Partridge L. Dietary restriction in long-lived dwarf flies. Science. 2002;296:319.
12. Curtsinger JW, Fukui HH, Townsend DR, Vaupel JW. Demography of genotypes: failure of the limited life-span paradigm in Drosophila melanogaster. Science. 1992;258:461–3.

13. Di Nicolantonio F, Martini M, Molinari F, Sartore-Bianchi A, Arena S, Saletti P, De DS, Mazzucchelli L, Frattini M, Siena S, Bardelli A. Wild-type BRAF is required for response to panitumumab or cetuximab in metastatic colorectal cancer. J Clin Oncol. 2008;26:5705–12.

14. Dotan E, Nicolas E, Devarajan K, Beck RJ, Cohen SJ. A pilot study evaluating peripheral blood lymphocyte telomere length in elderly versus young patients with colorectal cancer (CRC). In: 2012 Gastrointestinal cancers symposium. J Clin Oncol 30. 2012(suppl 4; abstr 512).

15. Douillard J, Siena S, Cassidy J, Tabernero J, Burkes R, Barugel ME, Humblet Y, Cunningham D, Wolf M, Gansert JL. Randomized phase 3 study of panitumumab with FOLFOX4 compared to FOLFOX4 alone as 1st-line treatment (tx) for metastatic colorectal cancer (mCRC): the PRIME trial. In: 2010 Gastrointestinal cancers symposium. Ann Oncol Supp. 2009.

16. Ewbank DC. Differences in the association between apolipoprotein E genotype and mortality across populations. J Gerontol A Biol Sci Med Sci. 2007;62:899–907.

17. Fearon ER, Vogelstein B. A genetic model for colorectal tumorigenesis. Cell. 1990;61: 759–67.

18. French AJ, Sargent DJ, Burgart LJ, Foster NR, Kabat BF, Goldberg R, Shepherd L, Windschitl HE, Thibodeau SN. Prognostic significance of defective mismatch repair and BRAF V600E in patients with colon cancer. Clin Cancer Res. 2008;14:3408–15.

19. Georgiades IB, Curtis LJ, Morris RM, Bird CC, Wyllie AH. Heterogeneity studies identify a subset of sporadic colorectal cancers without evidence for chromosomal or microsatellite instability. Oncogene. 1999;18:7933–40.

20. Gerdes LU, Jeune B, Ranberg KA, Nybo H, Vaupel JW. Estimation of apolipoprotein E genotype-specific relative mortality risks from the distribution of genotypes in centenarians and middle-aged men: apolipoprotein E gene is a "frailty gene," not a "longevity gene". Genet Epidemiol. 2000;19:202–10.

21. Greer EL, Dowlatshahi D, Banko MR, Villen J, Hoang K, Blanchard D, Gygi SP, Brunet A. An AMPK-FOXO pathway mediates longevity induced by a novel method of dietary restriction in C. elegans. Curr Biol. 2007;17:1646–56.

22. Hamilton WD. The moulding of senescence by natural selection. J Theor Biol. 1966;12: 12–45.

23. Harrison DE, Strong R, Sharp ZD, Nelson JF, Astle CM, Flurkey K, Nadon NL, Wilkinson JE, Frenkel K, Carter CS, Pahor M, Javors MA, Fernandez E, Miller RA. Rapamycin fed late in life extends lifespan in genetically heterogeneous mice. Nature. 2009;460:392–5.

24. Hecht JR, Mitchell E, Chidiac T, Scroggin C, Hagenstad C, Spigel D, Marshall J, Cohn A, McCollum D, Stella P, Deeter R, Shahin S, Amado RG. A randomized phase IIIB trial of chemotherapy, bevacizumab, and panitumumab compared with chemotherapy and bevacizumab alone for metastatic colorectal cancer. J Clin Oncol. 2009;27:672–80.

25. Hemminki A, Mecklin JP, Jarvinen H, Aaltonen LA, Joensuu H. Microsatellite instability is a favorable prognostic indicator in patients with colorectal cancer receiving chemotherapy. Gastroenterology. 2000;119:921–8.

26. Herndon LA, Schmeissner PJ, Dudaronek JM, Brown PA, Listner KM, Sakano Y, Paupard MC, Hall DH, Driscoll M. Stochastic and genetic factors influence tissue-specific decline in ageing C. elegans. Nature. 2002;419:808–14.

27. Honjoh S, Yamamoto T, Uno M, Nishida E. Signalling through RHEB-1 mediates intermittent fasting-induced longevity in C. elegans. Nature. 2009;457:726–30.

28. Issa JP. CpG island methylator phenotype in cancer. Nat Rev Cancer. 2004;4:988–93.

29. Kalaany NY, Sabatini DM. Tumours with PI3K activation are resistant to dietary restriction. Nature. 2009;458:725–31.

30. Kapahi P, Zid BM, Harper T, Koslover D, Sapin V, Benzer S. Regulation of lifespan in Drosophila by modulation of genes in the TOR signaling pathway. Curr Biol. 2004;14:885–90.

31. Karapetis CS, Khambata-Ford S, Jonker DJ, O'Callaghan CJ, Tu D, Tebbutt NC, Simes RJ, Chalchal H, Shapiro JD, Robitaille S, Price TJ, Shepherd L, Au HJ, Langer C, Moore MJ, Zalcberg JR. K-ras mutations and benefit from cetuximab in advanced colorectal cancer. N Engl J Med. 2008;359:1757–65.

32. Kenyon C. The plasticity of aging: insights from long-lived mutants. Cell. 2005;120:449–60.

33. Kenyon C, Chang J, Gensch E, Rudner A, Tabtiang R. A C. elegans mutant that lives twice as long as wild type. Nature. 1993;366:461–4.

34. Kenyon CJ. The genetics of ageing. Nature. 2010;464:504–12.

35. Li Y, Wang WJ, Cao H, Lu J, Wu C, Hu FY, Guo J, Zhao L, Yang F, Zhang YX, Li W, Zheng GY, Cui H, Chen X, Zhu Z, He H, Dong B, Mo X, Zeng Y, Tian XL. Genetic association of FOXO1A and FOXO3A with longevity trait in Han Chinese populations. Hum Mol Genet. 2009;18:4897–904.

36. Li Y, Xu W, McBurney MW, Longo VD. SirT1 inhibition reduces IGF-I/IRS-2/Ras/ERK1/2 signaling and protects neurons. Cell Metab. 2008;8:38–48.

37. Liang JT, Huang KC, Cheng AL, Jeng YM, Wu MS, Wang SM. Clinicopathological and molecular biological features of colorectal cancer in patients less than 40 years of age. Br J Surg. 2003;90:205–14.

38. Mair W, Goymer P, Pletcher SD, Partridge L. Demography of dietary restriction and death in Drosophila. Science. 2003;301:1731–3.

39. Oeppen J, Vaupel JW. Demography. Broken limits to life expectancy. Science. 2002;296: 1029–31.

40. Pawlikowska L, Hu D, Huntsman S, Sung A, Chu C, Chen J, Joyner AH, Schork NJ, Hsueh WC, Reiner AP, Psaty BM, Atzmon G, Barzilai N, Cummings SR, Browner WS, Kwok PY, Ziv E. Association of common genetic variation in the insulin/IGF1 signaling pathway with human longevity. Aging Cell. 2009;8:460–72.

41. Peyssonnaux C, Eychene A. The Raf/MEK/ERK pathway: new concepts of activation. Biol Cell. 2001;93:53–62.

42. Popat S, Hubner R, Houlston RS. Systematic review of microsatellite instability and colorectal cancer prognosis. J Clin Oncol. 2005;23:609–18.

43. Samowitz WS, Curtin K, Ma KN, Schaffer D, Coleman LW, Leppert M, Slattery ML. Microsatellite instability in sporadic colon cancer is associated with an improved prognosis at the population level. Cancer Epidemiol Biomarkers Prev. 2001;10:917–23.

44. Saridaki Z, Tzardi M, Papadaki C, Sfakianaki M, Pega F, Kalikaki A, Tsakalaki E, Trypaki M, Messaritakis I, Stathopoulos E, Mavroudis D, Georgoulias V, Souglakos J. Impact of KRAS, BRAF, PIK3CA mutations, PTEN, AREG, EREG expression and skin rash in >/= 2 line cetuximab-based therapy of colorectal cancer patients. PLoS One. 2011;6:e15980.

45. Sierra F, Hadley E, Suzman R, Hodes R. Prospects for life span extension. Annu Rev Med. 2009;60:457–69.

46. Souglakos J, Philips J, Wang R, Marwah S, Silver M, Tzardi M, Silver J, Ogino S, Hooshmand S, Kwak E, Freed E, Meyerhardt JA, Saridaki Z, Georgoulias V, Finkelstein D, Fuchs CS, Kulke MH, Shivdasani RA. Prognostic and predictive value of common mutations for treatment response and survival in patients with metastatic colorectal cancer. Br J Cancer. 2009;101: 465–72.

47. Tol J, Koopman M, Cats A, Rodenburg CJ, Creemers GJ, Schrama JG, Erdkamp FL, Vos AH, van Groeningen CJ, Sinnige HA, Richel DJ, Voest EE, Dijkstra JR, Vink-Borger ME, Antonini NF, Mol L, van Krieken JH, Dalesio O, Punt CJ. Chemotherapy, bevacizumab, and cetuximab in metastatic colorectal cancer. N Engl J Med. 2009;360:563–72.

48. Tomas-Loba A, Flores I, Fernandez-Marcos PJ, Cayuela ML, Maraver A, Tejera A, Borras C, Matheu A, Klatt P, Flores JM, Vina J, Serrano M, Blasco MA. Telomerase reverse transcriptase delays aging in cancer-resistant mice. Cell. 2008;135:609–22.

49. Van Cutsem E, Kohne CH, Hitre E, Zaluski J, Chang Chien CR, Makhson A, D'Haens G, Pinter T, Lim R, Bodoky G, Roh JK, Folprecht G, Ruff P, Stroh C, Tejpar S, Schlichting M, Nippgen J, Rougier P. Cetuximab and chemotherapy as initial treatment for metastatic colorectal cancer. N Engl J Med. 2009;360:1408–17.

50. Vaupel JW. Biodemography of human ageing. Nature. 2010;464:536–42.

51. Vaupel JW, Loichinger E. Redistributing work in aging Europe. Science. 2006;312:1911–3.

52. Vogelstein B, Kinzler KW. Cancer genes and the pathways they control. Nat Med. 2004;10: 789–99.

53. Wood LD, Parsons DW, Jones S, Lin J, Sjoblom T, Leary RJ, Shen D, Boca SM, Barber T, Ptak J, Silliman N, Szabo S, Dezso Z, Ustyanksky V, Nikolskaya T, Nikolsky Y, Karchin R, Wilson PA, Kaminker JS, Zhang Z, Croshaw R, Willis J, Dawson D, Shipitsin M, Willson JK, Sukumar S, Polyak K, Park BH, Pethiyagoda CL, Pant PV, Ballinger DG, Sparks AB, Hartigan J, Smith DR, Suh E, Papadopoulos N, Buckhaults P, Markowitz SD, Parmigiani G, Kinzler KW, Velculescu VE, Vogelstein B. The genomic landscapes of human breast and colorectal cancers. Science. 2007;318:1108–13.
54. Zbuk K, Sidebotham EL, Bleyer A, La Quaglia MP. Colorectal cancer in young adults. Semin Oncol. 2009;36:439–50.

Chapter 3
Comorbidity, Disability, and Geriatric Syndromes

Siri Rostoft Kristjansson

Abstract Comorbidity is defined as the presence of one or more disorders in addition to colorectal cancer. Comorbidity plays a role in a patient's individual risk of mortality and morbidity and may influence tolerance to cancer therapy. A comorbidity assessment is necessary to answer the following questions: Is the patient's remaining life expectancy likely to be limited by the colorectal cancer or by another comorbid medical condition? Will the comorbid condition(s) affect treatment tolerance? What are the interactions between the comorbid medical conditions and colorectal cancer?

Keywords Colorectal cancer • Frailty • Comorbidity • Geriatric assessment • Physiological reserves • Life expectancy • Competing risk • Older cancer patients • Geriatric syndromes

Comorbidity and Colorectal Cancer

Comorbidity is defined as the presence of one or more disorders in addition to colorectal cancer. Comorbidity plays a role in a patient's individual risk of mortality and morbidity and may influence tolerance to cancer therapy. A comorbidity assessment is necessary to answer the following questions: Is the patient's remaining life expectancy likely to be limited by the colorectal cancer or by another comorbid medical condition [1]? Will the comorbid condition(s) affect treatment tolerance? What are the interactions between the comorbid medical conditions and colorectal cancer?

S.R. Kristjansson, M.D., Ph.D.
Department of Internal Medicine,
Diakonhjemmet Hospital,
Diakonveien 12, Oslo 0319, Norway
e-mail: sirikristjansson@gmail.com

D. Papamichael, R.A. Audisio (eds.), *Management of Colorectal Cancers in Older People*,
DOI 10.1007/978-0-85729-984-0_3, © Springer-Verlag London 2013

The severity of comorbidity is associated with survival in cancer patients, independent of cancer stage [2]. Not surprisingly, it has been shown that the prognostic importance of overall comorbidity depends on the mortality burden of the index cancer: Comorbidities seem to have the greatest prognostic impact among groups with the highest survival rate and least impact in groups with the lowest survival rate [3]. In some cases, cancer treatment may do more harm than good if tumor complications are unlikely to occur during the patient's remaining lifetime. As previously mentioned, the majority of patients with colorectal cancer are older than 65 years. It has been estimated that the median number of comorbid conditions in older patients with colorectal cancer is four [4]. In a retrospective study based on cancer registry data, it was found that comorbidity had a substantial influence on colorectal cancer survival [4]. Approximately 18 % of deaths in the study cohort of 29,733 patients with a primary diagnosis of stage 1–3 colorectal cancer aged 67 years or older were attributable to chronic heart failure, chronic obstructive pulmonary disease, or diabetes mellitus. The authors point out that the effect of comorbidity is comparable with the effect of advanced-stage cancer because the predicted 5-year survival in a patients with stage I cancer and comorbidity was approximately 50 %. In comparison, the 5-year survival was approximately 78 % in an older patients with stage I cancer without comorbidity.

The influence of comorbidity on treatment and outcomes in older patients with cancer is not well understood. Some studies indicate that a few specific diseases matter [5], but the overall burden of disease may be even more important [6]. Unfortunately, in the majority of surgical publications, neither specific comorbidities nor the severity of comorbidities are registered preoperatively. Instead, American Society of Anesthesiologists physical status class (ASA class) is employed as a sole measure of comorbidity. ASA class only distinguishes between no systemic disease, mild systemic disease, and severe systemic disease. We will take a closer look at some studies that did measure comorbidity in older patients with colorectal cancer. Zingmond and colleagues studied predictors of serious medical and surgical complications after colorectal resections in 56,621 patients identified from the California hospital discharge database [7]. Independent predictors of serious medical complications were greater age, higher Charlson comorbidity index (CACI) score [8], and emergency surgery, while independent predictors of serious surgical complications were tumor location, greater age, and higher CACI score. Ouellette and colleagues evaluated CACI as a predictor of morbidity and mortality in 239 patients with colorectal carcinoma [9]. They found that CACI correlated with a longer length of stay, perioperative mortality, and overall mortality. However, in that study, CACI did not predict the severity of complications. In a retrospective registry study by Rabeneck and colleagues, 30-day mortality in older patients following surgery for colorectal carcinoma in the veteran affairs health-care system was studied [10]. On a side note, the multivariate analyses were not corrected for emergency versus elective procedures. The study found that predictors of 30-day mortality after rectal and colon cancer resections were age >65 years, comorbidity, and marital status. A study by Rutten and colleagues about total mesorectal excision and age used comorbidity data to show that comorbidity increased with increasing age up to 85–89 years, but they did not study the impact of comorbidity on postoperative morbidity or mortality [11]. Tan and colleagues studied a population of 121 octogenarians undergoing colorectal cancer surgery. In multivariate analyses, ASA class III and CACI scores over 5 were independent predictors of morbidity. Of note, only 13 (12.4 %) of their patients were ASA class III, and the majority of their octogenarians were actually ASA class I. In the preoperative assessment of cancer patients (PACE) study, the association between geriatric domains (activities of daily living (ADL), cognition, depression, and comorbidity), performance status, and fatigue and surgical outcomes in a sample of 460 older cancer patients was studied [12]. The majority of patients had breast cancer (47 %), while 31 % had colorectal cancer. PACE did not include nutritional data. Independent predictors of surgical morbidity were found to be fatigue and dependency in IADL. Comorbidity, measured by Satariano's index of comorbidities, did not predict postoperative morbidity. In a large study including 84,524 patients in France, 30-day postoperative mortality after CRC resection was independently associated with age 70 years or more, respiratory comorbidity, vascular comorbidity, neurologic comorbidity, emergency surgery, synchronous liver metastases, and preoperative malnutrition [13].

In summary, the available evidence clearly indicates that comorbidity is an independent contributing factor for adverse outcomes after CRC surgery, both when studying the comorbidity burden as well as independent comorbidities. Thus, all studies examining outcomes after CRC surgery should include data regarding comorbidity beyond ASA class. Furthermore, because comorbidity impacts on surgical mortality, morbidity, and survival, there is an obvious need to incorporate a pretreatment comorbidity assessment in all older patients with colorectal cancer.

Adjuvant chemotherapy is indicated in patients with stage III colon cancer in order to eradicate potential residual micrometastatic disease following surgical resection. It has been shown in numerous studies that the receipt of chemotherapy varies with age and comorbidity. Specific comorbidities that are associated with decreased likelihood of receiving chemotherapy are congestive heart failure, chronic obstructive pulmonary disease, and diabetes [14]. More studies looking at the impact of comorbidity on receipt of chemotherapy and chemotherapy toxicity in this patient population are warranted.

Disability and Geriatric Syndromes

In older patients in general, optimizing functional status is one of the major treatment goals. This is also important in all phases of care of older patients with cancer. Being hospitalized is an event that frequently precipitates disability [15]. However, surgical studies dealing with treatment for CRC in older patients rarely include information about preoperative physical function or the adverse effect of surgery on physical function. The most commonly used outcome measures in the surgical literature are postoperative mortality, postoperative morbidity, and survival – thus disregarding one of the main treatment goals: optimizing functional status. It has been shown that seriously ill patients are willing to undergo burdensome treatment for the sake of survival, but not if the consequence is disability or cognitive decline [16]. About one-third of patients older than 70 years of age experience hospitalization-associated disability (defined as the loss of ability to complete one of the basic ADLs needed to live independently: bathing, dressing, rising from a bed or chair, using the toilet, eating, or walking across a room). In clinical practice, the recognition of limitations in functional status is mandatory in order to prevent and manage disability postoperatively. Furthermore, functional status is a powerful predictor of postoperative outcomes [6, 9, 12, 17–19]. Measuring preoperative functional status is particularly important in older surgical patients, where the proportion of patients with disabilities is higher than in younger patient cohorts. Furthermore, functional status is one of the most powerful predictors of survival in general [20] and thus need to be incorporated in an overall treatment plan weighing risks and benefits for cancer patients.

The long-term effects of treatment for CRC on disability have been evaluated in population-based studies. Hewitt and colleagues found that cancer survivors in general were more likely to report limitations of ADLs or instrumental ADLs and functional disabilities than individuals without a history of cancer [21]. This effect was less evident for men with a history of CRC. Lawrence and colleagues studied the effect of abdominal surgery on functional status [22]. They found that potentially modifiable independent predictors of ADL and IADL recovery were preoperative physical conditioning and depression, in addition to serious postoperative complications. The clinical course of functional recovery varied across different measures, and protracted disability at 6 months after operation was substantial.

The term "geriatric syndromes" is used by geriatricians to highlight the unique features of health conditions that are commonly seen in older people. Examples of geriatric syndromes are falls, frailty, functional decline, delirium, and incontinence. These syndromes are difficult to capture in established disease categories. For research purposes, the concept of geriatric syndromes is still poorly defined. A common feature of geriatric syndromes is that they are multifactorial [23]. Multiple organ systems are involved, and the chief complaint may not necessarily involve the site of the physiological insult. Instead, the symptoms arise from the organ with the least physiological reserves. This may be illustrated with a clinical example commonly seen: An older patient develops delirium because of a urinary tract infection (UTI). Even though the pathology is located in the bladder, the patient presents with disorganized thinking and inattention instead of frequent and painful voiding. Delirium in the course of an infection or after surgery is often seen in patients with limited cognitive reserves. Delirium cannot be explained by a single cause (UTI), but it occurs because the patient has impairments in multiple domains. Due to impairments such as comorbidities, cognitive impairment, and limited social support, the patient is vulnerable, and the UTI may be viewed as a precipitating event that then triggers the syndrome of delirium. This way of thinking is useful for understanding how to prevent disability and geriatric syndromes in older patients undergoing treatment for CRC. Surgery and subsequent hospitalization lead to functional loss, and several factors contribute to this negative spiral. A first step for successful prevention is the identification of pretreatment determinants of vulnerability, such as higher age (especially age over 85 years), poor mobility, comorbidity, cognitive dysfunction, dependency in ADLs and IADLs, depression, and geriatric syndromes. These factors are assessed through a geriatric assessment (Chap. 5). The next step is to minimize the surgical trauma, for example, through the enhanced recovery after surgery (ERAS) principles proposed by Kehlet and colleagues [24], or by choosing minimally invasive surgery when possible. Postoperatively, factors such as early ambulation, early nutrition, and early return to home may facilitate recovery. It is important to avoid enforced dependence, a disturbing environment (distortion of the night-day cycle, frequent personnel changes, noisy environment), and polypharmacy. A planned discharge from the hospital is easier when an *early assessment* of post-discharge needs is performed, thus avoiding a rushed planning immediately before discharge, which increases the risk of overlooking important factors that may contribute to rehospitalization.

Frailty is a geriatric syndrome that attracts special attention from researchers and clinicians who deal with older patients. Frailty describes "an elderly patient who is at heightened vulnerability to adverse health status change because of a multisystem reduction in reserve capacity," but after years of debate, it remains controversial how to identify frailty in an individual patient [25]. Treatment modalities such as surgery and chemotherapy put a cancer patient at risk of complications and toxicity, and identifying frailty is thus particularly important in older patients with cancer. Within geriatric oncology, a frailty definition derived from criteria first described by Winograd and later modified by Balducci has been proposed [26]. Based on a geriatric assessment (GA), an older adult is considered frail when fulfilling any of the following criteria: dependency in activities of daily living (ADL), three or more comorbid illnesses, the presence of geriatric syndromes (e.g., dementia, malnutrition, depression, delirium, and falls), or age >85 years. This may be considered a multicomponent phenotype of frailty, and deficits across different health domains, such as clinical, psychological, and functional, are expected to predict treatment tolerance and life expectancy. Rockwood and colleagues have proposed an approach to defining frailty where accumulation of deficits is counted. The more deficits you have, the frailer you are [27]. In Rockwood's definition, a frailty index is constructed based on a GA [28]. Within the geriatric and biogerontological literature, a widely accepted definition of frailty is based on data from more than 5,000 community dwelling individuals aged 65 years and older who participated in the cardiovascular health study [29]. The physical phenotype of frailty (PF) is defined as fulfilling at least three of the following five criteria: unintentional weight loss, exhaustion, slow walking speed, low physical activity, and weakness. This approach to defining frailty disregards comorbidity and cognition. A physiologic loss of reserves is identified through clusters of physical impairments. PF predicts incident falls, hospitalizations, worsening mobility, and deaths in large cohorts [29, 30]. Two studies have looked at whether PF predicts postoperative complications after CRC surgery, and the results were conflicting [31, 32]. To my knowledge, no studies have specifically studied the impact of PF on chemotherapy toxicity in older patients with CRC.

Dementia is a geriatric syndrome that impacts delivery of care for CRC. Little data is available, but a few studies have specifically investigated how a diagnosis of dementia influences CRC diagnosis, treatment, and survival. In one study, based on cancer registry data, patients with a mental disorder had a greater likelihood of being diagnosed at an unknown stage or being diagnosed at autopsy [33]. Thirteen percent of patients with a diagnosis of dementia in that study did not receive any treatment for their CRC, and for patients with stage III CRC, 79 % did not receive adjuvant chemotherapy. Less than 10 % of the patients in the study had dementia, and registry data must be interpreted with caution because dementia is under diagnosed in the elderly. In another study from 2004, also based on cancer registry data from the USA, Gupta and colleagues reported that patients with dementia were twice as likely to be diagnosed with colon cancer after death [34]. They also found that patients with stage I to III disease were half as likely to undergo surgical resection for their colon carcinoma.

Conclusion

For older patients with CRC, there is a large body of evidence indicating that comorbidity, disability, and geriatric syndromes impact on diagnosis, treatment, toxicity, morbidity, and survival. If these factors are not taken into consideration, there is a risk of both overtreatment and under-treatment. A geriatric assessment involves these important patient factors and allows for individualized treatment decisions.

References

1. Welch HG, Albertsen PC, Nease RF, Bubolz TA, Wasson JH. Estimating treatment benefits for the elderly: the effect of competing risks. Ann Intern Med. 1996;124(6):577–84.
2. Piccirillo JF, Tierney RM, Costas I, Grove L, Spitznagel Jr EL. Prognostic importance of comorbidity in a hospital-based cancer registry. JAMA. 2004;291(20):2441–7.
3. Read WL, Tierney RM, Page NC, et al. Differential prognostic impact of comorbidity. J Clin Oncol. 2004;22(15):3099–103.
4. Gross CP, Guo Z, McAvay GJ, Allore HG, Young M, Tinetti ME. Multimorbidity and survival in older persons with colorectal cancer. J Am Geriatr Soc. 2006;54(12):1898–904.
5. Lemmens VE, Janssen-Heijnen ML, Houterman S, et al. Which comorbid conditions predict complications after surgery for colorectal cancer? World J Surg. 2007;31(1):192–9.
6. Kristjansson SR, Jordhøy MS, Nesbakken A, et al. Which elements of a comprehensive geriatric assessment (CGA) predict post-operative complications and early mortality after colorectal cancer surgery? J Geriatr Oncol. 2010;1(2):57–65.
7. Zingmond D, Maggard M, O'Connell J, Liu J, Etzioni D, Ko C. What predicts serious complications in colorectal cancer resection? Am Surg. 2003;69(11):969–74.
8. Charlson ME, Pompei P, Ales KL, MacKenzie CR. A new method of classifying prognostic comorbidity in longitudinal studies: development and validation. J Chronic Dis. 1987;40(5):373–83.
9. Ouellette JR, Small DG, Termuhlen PM. Evaluation of Charlson-Age Comorbidity Index as predictor of morbidity and mortality in patients with colorectal carcinoma. J Gastrointest Surg. 2004;8(8):1061–7.
10. Rabeneck L, Davila JA, Thompson M, El-Serag HB. Outcomes in elderly patients following surgery for colorectal cancer in the veterans affairs health care system. Aliment Pharmacol Ther. 2004;20(10):1115–24.

11. Rutten HJ, den Dulk M, Lemmens VE, van de Velde CJ, Marijnen CA. Controversies of total mesorectal excision for rectal cancer in elderly patients. Lancet Oncol. 2008;9(5):494–501.
12. Audisio RA, Pope D, Ramesh HS, et al. Shall we operate? Preoperative assessment in elderly cancer patients (PACE) can help. A SIOG surgical task force prospective study. Crit Rev Oncol Hematol. 2008;65(2):156–63.
13. Panis Y, Maggiori L, Caranhac G, Bretagnol F, Vicaut E. Mortality after colorectal cancer surgery: a French survey of more than 84,000 patients. Ann Surg. 2011;254(5):738–43; discussion 743–4.
14. Gross CP, McAvay GJ, Krumholz HM, Paltiel AD, Bhasin D, Tinetti ME. The effect of age and chronic illness on life expectancy after a diagnosis of colorectal cancer: implications for screening. Ann Intern Med. 2006;145(9):646–53.
15. Covinsky KE, Pierluissi E, Johnston CB. Hospitalization-associated disability: "she was probably able to ambulate, but I'm not sure". JAMA. 2011;306(16):1782–93.
16. Fried TR, Bradley EH, Towle VR, Allore H. Understanding the treatment preferences of seriously ill patients. N Engl J Med. 2002;346(14):1061–6.
17. Sunouchi K, Namiki K, Mori M, Shimizu T, Tadokoro M. How should patients 80 years of age or older with colorectal carcinoma be treated? Long-term and short-term outcome and postoperative cytokine levels. Dis Colon Rectum. 2000;43(2):233–41.
18. Gurevitch AJ, Davidovitch B, Kashtan H. Outcome of right colectomy for cancer in octogenarians. J Gastrointest Surg. 2009;13(1):100–4.
19. Hamel MB, Henderson WG, Khuri SF, Daley J. Surgical outcomes for patients aged 80 and older: morbidity and mortality from major noncardiac surgery. J Am Geriatr Soc. 2005;53(3):424–9.
20. Walter LC, Brand RJ, Counsell SR, et al. Development and validation of a prognostic index for 1-year mortality in older adults after hospitalization. JAMA. 2001;285(23):2987–94.
21. Hewitt M, Rowland JH, Yancik R. Cancer survivors in the United States: age, health, and disability. J Gerontol A Biol Sci Med Sci. 2003;58(1):82–91.
22. Lawrence VA, Hazuda HP, Cornell JE, et al. Functional independence after major abdominal surgery in the elderly. J Am Coll Surg. 2004;199(5):762–72.
23. Inouye SK, Studenski S, Tinetti ME, Kuchel GA. Geriatric syndromes: clinical, research, and policy implications of a core geriatric concept. J Am Geriatr Soc. 2007;55(5):780–91.
24. Kehlet H. Fast-track colorectal surgery. Lancet. 2008;371(9615):791–3.
25. Martin FC, Brighton P. Frailty: different tools for different purposes? Age Ageing. 2008;37(2):129–31.
26. Balducci L, Extermann M. Management of cancer in the older person: a practical approach. Oncologist. 2000;5(3):224–37.
27. Rockwood K, Mitnitski A. Frailty in relation to the accumulation of deficits. J Gerontol A Biol Sci Med Sci. 2007;62(7):722–7.
28. Jones DM, Song X, Rockwood K. Operationalizing a frailty index from a standardized comprehensive geriatric assessment. J Am Geriatr Soc. 2004;52(11):1929–33.
29. Fried LP, Tangen CM, Walston J, et al. Frailty in older adults: evidence for a phenotype. J Gerontol A Biol Sci Med Sci. 2001;56(3):M146–56.
30. Ensrud KE, Ewing SK, Taylor BC, et al. Frailty and risk of falls, fracture, and mortality in older women: the study of osteoporotic fractures. J Gerontol A Biol Sci Med Sci. 2007;62(7):744–51.
31. Kristjansson SR, Ronning B, Hurria A, Skovlund E, Jordhøy MS, Nesbakken A, Wyller TB. A comparison of two pre-operative frailty measures in older surgical cancer patients. J Geriatr Oncol. 2012;3(1):1–7.
32. Tan KY, Kawamura YJ, Tokomitsu A, Tang T. Assessment for frailty is useful for predicting morbidity in elderly patients undergoing colorectal cancer resection whose comorbidities are already optimized. Am J Surg. 2012;204(2):139–43.
33. Baillargeon J, Kuo YF, Lin YL, Raji MA, Singh A, Goodwin JS. Effect of mental disorders on diagnosis, treatment, and survival of older adults with colon cancer. J Am Geriatr Soc. 2011;59(7):1268–73.
34. Gupta SK, Lamont EB. Patterns of presentation, diagnosis, and treatment in older patients with colon cancer and comorbid dementia. J Am Geriatr Soc. 2004;52(10):1681–7.

Chapter 4
CRC: Diagnosis, Staging, and Patient Assessment

Siri Rostoft Kristjansson and Riccardo A. Audisio

Abstract Colorectal cancer often presents as an emergency with signs of obstruction, poor general conditions [1, 2]. This is associated with high mortality, increased complication rate [3], and a poor oncologic result [4]. This is particularly relevant to older patients. Every effort should be put in place to avoid the emergency setting. To achieve this, screening programs have been put in place.

Keywords Preoperative assessment • Comorbidity • Operative risk • Risk prediction • Cancer surgery • Elderly

Introduction

Colorectal cancer often presents as an emergency with signs of obstruction, poor general conditions [1, 2]. This is associated with high mortality, increased complication rate [3], and a poor oncologic result [4]. This is particularly relevant to older patients. Every effort should be put in place to avoid the emergency setting. To achieve this, screening programs have been put in place.

S.R. Kristjansson, M.D., Ph.D.
Department of Internal Medicine, Diakonhjemmet Hospital,
Diakonveien 12, 0319 Oslo, Norway

R.A. Audisio, M.D., FRCS (✉)
Department of Surgery, St. Helens and Knowsley Teaching Hospitals,
Marshalls Cross Road, St Helens, Merseyside WA9 3DA, UK
e-mail: raudisio@doctors.org.uk

D. Papamichael, R.A. Audisio (eds.), *Management of Colorectal Cancers in Older People*, 29
DOI 10.1007/978-0-85729-984-0_4, © Springer-Verlag London 2013

Screening

So far, colorectal cancer is not entirely preventable; modifications in diet and lifestyle should substantially reduce the risk of the disease and could complement screening in reducing colorectal cancer incidence. Secondary prevention has thus been considered to reduce the large bowel cancer death. Older people are at greater risk of many types of cancer than other age groups but those with a low life expectancy are unlikely to benefit from screening, as even if screening detects a malignancy, they may not live long enough for it to manifest clinically. It is important to remember that there is great variation in individual health status with increasing age, so in an elderly population screening, decisions made on an individual basis are increasingly important.

The British Geriatric Society [5] has proposed a screening framework [6] to be used to guide screening decisions in older individuals. This framework takes into account life expectancy, risk of dying from screen-detectable cancers, and the risks and benefits of the screening tests, as well as the individual's situation and preferences. This model is more appropriate than defining an age at which screening should be stopped, as older people of the same age may vary greatly in terms of life expectancy and personal screening preferences.

The UK NHS Bowel Screening Programme [7] currently offers screening every 2 years to everyone aged 60–69. An explanatory letter and fecal occult blood test (FOBT) testing kit is sent by post, and results are reported within 2 weeks. People over 70 can request a kit, but are not sent one automatically. People with a positive FOBT, without any other likely causes for this result (e.g., known bowel pathology, dietary or pharmacological causes), are referred for colonoscopy. People with an unclear FOBT result should repeat the test. Everyone who has an abnormal result after completing the screening test for bowel cancer will be invited to discuss having a colonoscopy.

At present patients are sent information by post about screening and how to attend. An age extension up to age 75 was agreed and recently confirmed by the coalition government and is presently being set in place (five screening centers started implementing the age extension in 2008). As screening centers complete their first 2-year screening round, they are rolling out the extension (subject to meeting criteria and subsequent approval by the national office). By October 2011, 32 of the 58 local screening centers had started inviting the extended population.

Several large randomized controlled studies have been carried out which provide evidence that screening with FOBT every other year significantly reduces colorectal cancer mortality [8].

However, screening is not 100 % effective in preventing deaths from cancer. Screening may miss very early stage disease and may also detect some disease which is too advanced to be treatable. Screening may also detect cancer which may never have produced clinical symptoms if the patient has other comorbidities which result in death before the disease progresses. Walter and Covinsky [6] explain that even if screening is effective in early detection of disease, it is unlikely to benefit people with low life expectancies as the benefits of screening, that is, increased survival from cancer, are not significant until at least 5 years after the start of screening, for the current cancer screening programs. They go on to explain that this time may be even greater than 5 years in people over 70 as "some evidence suggests that the length of time that a screen-detectable cancer remains clinically asymptomatic increases with advancing age for both breast and colorectal cancer." The reason for the time interval between screening and survival benefit is because it is generally only the early presymptomatic cancers which benefit from earlier treatment. Thus, screening is probably not appropriate for people with life expectancies of less than 5 years.

Besides the advantage of detecting colorectal cancers at an early stage, screening tests pose some potentially harmful effects. It is important to remember that a screening test will benefit only a small percentage of the people having the test but expose all to the risks. Risks of screening fall into four main categories:

1. Complications from the tests themselves – for example, colonoscopy carries a risk of bowel perforation.
2. Unnecessary treatment for cancers which would never have become symptomatic or presented clinically at all. As life expectancy decreases, the probability that a cancer which is detected will never be clinically significant increases.
3. Anxiety and psychological harms from either the testing process itself or from being given a false-positive result.
4. Patients being overly reassured by a negative result and therefore not reporting symptoms to their GP/geriatrician.

There has been little research on screening in older people, and few current guidelines recommend an upper age limit for screening. The UK Colorectal Cancer Screening Pilot, which led to the introduction of the NHS Bowel Screening Programme, excluded people over 70 years of age because of a falloff in uptake over this age in the Nottingham trial of FOBT screening [9]. In the Danish trial of fecal occult blood screening [10], 25 % of detectable cancers would have been missed if an age cutoff of 69 years (as chosen for the England program) rather than 74 years had been used.

There are therefore several issues to be considered in developing cancer screening guidelines for older people:

The safety of screening tests – is there an age at which the risks of intervention outweigh the benefits that may be gained?

Is life expectancy a more meaningful criterion to decide whether to offer a test than simply age?

Should a series of negative screening tests mean that further tests are unnecessary or can be delayed? This has already been done for cervical screening, but not for colorectal screening programs.

The British Geriatric Society [5] has therefore proposed a model of screening older patients for cancer on the assumption that life expectancy is more important in guiding screening decisions than actual age, as life expectancy varies widely between people of the same age, depending on their comorbid conditions. Hence "an 85-year-old woman in the upper quartile of life expectancy has more chance of benefiting from cancer screening than a 75-year-old woman in the lower quartile" [6].

It was recommended that a conceptual "screening framework," similar to that proposed by Walter and Covinsky [6], be used to guide individual screening decisions, rather than a rigid set of age-specific guidelines. This framework entails four key steps:

Step 1: Estimate the patient's risk of dying of a screening-detectable cancer. This risk is estimated first by knowing the age-specific mortality rate of the cancer and then the person's life expectancy. So if life expectancy is estimated at 5 years, and the cancer in question's age-specific annual mortality is 200 deaths in 100,000, then the deaths attributable to that cancer are $5 \times 200/100,000 = 1$ %. The Office for National Statistics produces cohort life expectancy tables [14] which are calculated using age-specific mortality rates and take into account predicted changes in mortality in the future. They are regarded as a better measure of how many more years a person of a particular age is likely to live for than period life expectancy calculations. At present, 2008 UK statistics show that men aged 88 in 2010 had a life expectancy of over 5 years (5.2 years) and women aged 89 in 2010 had a life expectancy of over 5 years (5.3 years).

The geriatrician will need to use known variables such as number and severity of comorbid conditions and functional status to estimate whether a person's life expectancy is in the middle, upper, or lower quartiles of their age-sex cohort.

Step 2: Next, the possible outcomes of screening tests need to be considered. For example, if this person has a positive FOBT, would further investigation with colonoscopy be appropriate? If not, then there is little point in carrying out FOBT, as a positive result is likely to generate anxiety without offering any later reassurance or intervention. Then, the potential for benefit if treatment is given needs to be considered – not every cancer will be curatively treated. Trials data combined with the likelihood of dying from a cancer (rather than something else) reveals the number needed to be screened (NNS) to save one life from dying of that cancer. For breast and colon cancer, the NNS rises with age beyond 70.

Step 3: The harm of cancer screening needs to be considered. While psychological harm may be similar at all ages, the risks of certain investigations rise with age.

Step 4: Finally, and most importantly, the risks and benefits of screening need to be weighed up with the individual's situation and preferences, determined by the patient's view of ageing and mortality.

The actual screening test used is the same at all ages. The risks and benefits of each test should be clearly explained to people before they undergo the tests. Ideally this would be done by a GP or geriatrician on an individual basis.

The geriatrician's or GP's role in screening is to guide the patient toward making the right decision. This involves using their clinical knowledge of the patient's comorbidities and physical examination to estimate life expectancy; using their knowledge of screening procedures to explain the risks and benefits of screening, including the risks and benefits of declining screening tests; and using their personal knowledge of the patient's preferences and values in helping the patient to come to an informed decision about screening.

Research shows that physicians often do not take into account the impact that higher rates of comorbidity and disability in elderly people may have on the risks and benefits of screening tests for them. A 2006 survey of over 2,000 physicians revealed that when presented with "case scenarios" of patients aged 70, 80, or 90 and with differing comorbidities, most factored life expectancy into their decision about screening advice for the patient. However, over 30 % indicated a "high likelihood" of offering a frail 90-year-old a mammogram, and 13.4 % would offer this person cervical screening. The tendency to "overscreen" elderly people with under 5 years median life expectancy was greater than the tendency to "underscreen" elderly people with over 10 years median life expectancy [11].

The patient's own preferences are the final step in the proposed framework in coming to a decision about screening. In the context of cognitive decline, understanding of the risks and benefits, and the relief at a negative screening test, may be diminished, while anxiety in relation to tests may be increased. In these cases the geriatrician may play an important role in presenting the information about screening in such a way that the patient's ability to make their own decision is optimized and if this is not possible, perhaps in discussing the issue with family members as part of the decision-making process.

The geriatrician and the general practitioner may both play an important role in explaining the testing procedures and risks and benefits to patients. The English Bowel Cancer Screening Pilot [7] studies involved inviting 478, 250 people aged 50–69 for screening, and the uptake of FOBT was 56.8 %. Thirteen percent of people said they wanted much more information before considering screening [12]. This indicates that better explanations of the tests are needed, and geriatricians would be well placed to do this.

British Geriatric Society's recommendations:

Older people should not be excluded from national cancer screening programmes.

It recommends that screening be offered to those over 70 with an estimated life-expectancy of over 5 years. Older people with life-expectancies of less than 5 years are unlikely to benefit from cancer screening.

Screening should be considered on an individualized basis. General Practitioners should discuss screening with their patients, using their knowledge of the comorbidities (and therefore likely life expectancy) as well as the patient's preferences and views. They should assist the patient in coming to an informed decision. GPs could refer individual patients onto Geriatricians if they feel any more detailed discussions are necessary at any stage of the screening process.

The age at which cancer screening is beneficial is likely to rise as investigations become safer and more predictive, and life expectancy increases. Age cutoffs for national programmes should be constantly reviewed with this in mind.

At present there is some evidence that cervical screening is not recommended in elderly people who have had several consecutive previous negative tests, as the incidence of disease in these people is very low.

Diagnosis

As in the younger age groups, it is recommended that suspected cancers of the colon and rectum should be confirmed by an endoscopic procedure (colonoscopy or sigmoidoscopy) and tissue sampling.

Confirmed cancers of the colon should be staged with a CT of the chest and abdomen; when this is not feasible, a chest x-ray and an ultrasound scan of the abdomen should be taken to stage the extent of the disease.

An MRI is often helpful for patients presenting with pelvic lesions, in order to assess nodal involvement as well as defining the local extent of the disease.

Virtual colonoscopy (also called computerized tomographic colonography – CTC) is used to produce pictures of the colon and rectum. A computer then assembles these pictures into detailed images that can show polyps and other abnormalities. Because it is less invasive than standard colonoscopy and sedation is not needed, virtual colonoscopy may cause less discomfort and take less time to perform. As with standard colonoscopy, a thorough cleansing of the colon is necessary before this test. Furthermore, CTC does not allow for tissue sampling. Whether virtual colonoscopy can reduce the number of deaths from colorectal cancer is not yet known, but it was suggested that implementing a program of 5-yearly CTC as a primary screen is expected to be more expensive than FOBT screening over the short term, despite substantial savings in treatment costs over the 10-year time horizon [13]. Advocates of this procedure suggest how limited-preparation low-dose CTC is a feasible and useful minimally invasive technique with which to evaluate the colon and exclude gross pathology (mass lesions and polyps >1 cm) in elderly patients with diminished performance status, yielding good to excellent image quality [14].

Although the ability of CTC to demonstrate polyps <6 mm is limited, the clinical significance of detecting 5 mm and smaller polyps is questionable. Fifty percent of colonic polyps ≤5 mm are nonneoplastic, and less than 2 % of all polyps ≤5 mm have advanced histology [15, 16].

A decision analysis of the relative yield of referring patients with polyps ≤5 mm to colonoscopic polypectomy demonstrated that 562 such polyps would have to be removed to avoid leaving behind one advanced adenoma. Thus, colonoscopy referral for polyps ≤5 mm likely would do more harm than good, as it would prove to be very costly and would introduce many unnecessary complications especially in the older population [17].

Patient Assessment

Colorectal cancer surgery in the elderly has been addressed in a number of surgical publications in the last years. Already in 1980, Boyd and colleagues elegantly showed that mortality rates after colon resection (70 % of the patients had colon cancer) compared by decades of age correlated with the number of preexisting conditions and not with age as an isolated factor [18]. They concluded that a careful preoperative assessment, correction of preexisting pulmonary and nutritional deficiencies, and avoidance of emergency procedures might improve morbidity and mortality rates associated with colon resections in elderly patients. A large systematic review published in 2000 looked at how the outcomes of surgery for colorectal cancer differed between elderly and younger patients [19]. The cohort consisted of

34,194 patients and was divided into the following age groups: aged less than 65 years, aged 65–74 years, aged 75–84 years, and aged 85+ years. Postoperative morbidity and mortality were found to increase with age. The authors proposed that this could be attributed to the following factors being more common with advancing age: comorbidity, the rate of emergency operations, and the rate of advanced cancer stages. They also found that elderly patients were less likely to undergo curative surgery. Overall survival was poorer for the older patients, but the differences in cancer-specific survival were less noticeable. A recent study from English NHS hospitals including 28,746 elective colorectal cancer resections in patients >75 years found that increasing age was an independent predictor of 30-day mortality and 1-year mortality [20]. This study was based on registry data, and comorbidity data were available. Functional status was unfortunately not included in the analyses in that study.

When studying the surgical literature regarding the impact of increasing age on surgical outcomes, a direct comparison between published studies is complicated because of methodological differences. Most studies lack information about potentially important patient variables such as comorbidity, functional status, nutritional status, and cognitive function. When the outcome is postoperative complications, there are differences between methods of recording and scoring of morbidity that make results incomparable. In most studies, comorbidity beyond ASA score, functional status, and nutritional status are found to be independent predictors of postoperative mortality and morbidity when they are included in preoperative risk models in older patients undergoing CRC surgery [20–24]. Another problem when comparing results from individual trials is that the outcomes after colorectal cancer surgery are highly influenced by perioperative variables. For example, it has been demonstrated that an enhanced recovery after surgery program (ERAS) for elective bowel surgery may reduce morbidity, lead to a faster recovery, and shorten hospital stay [25]. This accelerated multimodal rehabilitation program includes, among other factors, optimal pain relief, stress reduction with regional anesthesia, early enteral nutrition, and early mobilization. Another strategy that was recently shown to improve surgical quality was the implementation of surgical checklists during different phases of perioperative care [26]. Furthermore, there are now several indications that older patients undergoing laparoscopic CRC surgery have favorable outcomes compared to patients undergoing open surgery [20, 27]. In summary, when studying risk factors for negative postoperative outcomes in older patients undergoing CRC surgery, there are several pre-, intra-, and postoperative factors that need to be elucidated, and to date there are no "one size fits all" data.

In CRC, surgery is often inevitable because the tumor itself poses a direct risk of complications such as bleeding, obstruction, or perforation. As emergency surgery carries a substantially higher risk than elective surgery, even more pronounced in older patients, a planned surgical procedure is recommended. A preoperative risk assessment based on ASA class or the colorectal cancer model of the Association of Coloproctology of Great Britain and Ireland provides some information about the risk of postoperative mortality, but in elective CRC surgery, this risk rarely exceed about 5 %, even in cohorts consisting of older adults only. A more interesting approach in these patients is to use preoperative tools that provide information beyond the surgical risk. It has been suggested to use tools from a geriatric assessment (GA) to assess older patients before CRC surgery. Areas where older adults often present with problems are systematically assessed. The general composition of a GA involves functional status, comorbidity, polypharmacy, nutritional status, cognitive function, emotional status, and social support. Recent publications have found that elements from a GA independently predict postoperative outcomes in older CRC patients [21, 28]. There are several arguments favoring completing a GA as a preoperative assessment in older adults. Firstly, GA may uncover previously unknown medical problems, such as cognitive dysfunction and depression. Cognitive problems necessitate adjustments of the preoperative counseling, have implications for choice of treatment, and increase the risk of postoperative delirium, which may be prevented. Secondly, knowledge about social support, functional status, and cognition may provide information about adherence to treatment protocol. In some cases, arrangements must be made regarding transportation and emergency contacts. It is also possible that preoperative interventions based on a GA, such as optimization of comorbidity and malnutrition and improved functional status through specific exercise regimens, may reduce postoperative complication rates. Clinical trials investigating this are ongoing.

Conclusion

Despite the modest amount of evidence available on screening for CRC in older patients, every effort should be made toward the detection of colorectal malignancies at an early stage. Computerized tomographic colonography is well tolerated and worth considering due to the minimally intrusive bowel preparation required.

Frailty assessment is mandatory; it will guide the clinicians on diagnosis, staging, and treatment plans. More on, it will allow active pre-habilitation and correction of malnourishment, anemia, dehydration, and depression; these conditions associate to a poorer outcome, higher complications rate, mortality, and higher costs.

References

1. Cheynel N, Cortet M, Lepage C, Benoit L, Faivre J, Bouvier AM. Trends in frequency and management of obstructing colorectal cancers in a well-defined population. Dis Colon Rectum. 2007;50(10):1568–75.
2. Tekkis PP, Kinsman R, Thompson MR, Stamatakis JD. The Association of Coloproctology of Great Britain and Ireland study of large bowel obstruction caused by colorectal cancer. Ann Surg. 2004;240(1):76–81.
3. Sjo O, Larsen S, Lunde O, Nesbakken A. Short term outcome after emergency and elective surgery for colon cancer. Colorectal Dis. 2008;11(7):733–9.

4. Ohman U. Prognosis in patients with obstructing colorectal carcinoma. Am J Surg. 1982;143(6):742–7.

5. http://www.bgs.org.uk/index.php?option=com_content&view=article&id=1176:canceroldpeo ple&catid=12:goodpractice&Itemid=106.

6. Walter LC, Covinsky KE. Cancer screening in elderly patients: a framework for individualized decision making. JAMA. 2001;285(21):2750–6.

7. NHS Bowel Cancer Screening Programme. www.cancerscreening.nhs.uk/bowel/. Last accessed 24 November 2012.

8. Anwar S, Hall C, Elder JB. Screening for colorectal cancer: present, past and future. Eur J Surg Oncol. 1998;24:477–86.

9. Population screening for colorectal cancer. Drug Ther Bull. 2006;44(9):65–8.

10. Kronborg O, Fenger C, Olsen J, et al. Randomised study of screening for colorectal cancer with faecal-occult-blood test. Lancet. 1996;348:1467–71.

11. Heflin MT, et al. The impact of health status on physicians' intentions to offer cancer screening to older women. J Gerontol A Biol Sci Med Sci. 2006;61(8):844–50.

12. Information from and about the screening programme http://www.cancerscreening.nhs.uk/ bowel/programme-information.html. Last accessed 24 November 2012.

13. Keighley MRB. Screening for colorectal cancer in Europe. Scand J Gastroenterol. 2004;9:805–6.

14. Sweet A, Lee D, Gairy K, Phiri D, Reason T, Lock K. The impact of CT colonography for colorectal cancer screening on the UK NHS: costs, healthcare resources and health outcomes. Appl Health Econ Health Policy. 2011;9(1):51–64.

15. Keeling AN, Slattery MM, Leong S, McCarthy E, Susanto M, Lee MJ, Morrin MM. Limited-preparation CT colonography in frail elderly patients: a feasibility study. AJR Am J Roentgenol. 2010 May;194(5):1279–87.

16. Lieberman D, Moravec M, Holub J, Michaels L, Eisen G. Polyp size and advanced histology in patients undergoing colonoscopy screening: implications for CT colonography. Gastroenterology. 2008;135:1100–5.

17. Butterly LF, Chase MP, Pohl H, Fiarman GS. Prevalence of clinically important histology in small adenomas. Clin Gastroenterol Hepatol. 2006;4:343–8.

18. http://www.ncbi.nlm.nih.gov/pubmed/19965295.

19. Boyd JB, Bradford Jr B, Watne AL. Operative risk factors of colon resection in the elderly. Ann Surg. 1980;192(6):743–6.

20. Surgery for colorectal cancer in elderly patients: a systematic review. Colorectal Cancer Collaborative Group. Lancet. 2000;356(9234):968–74.

21. Faiz O, Haji A, Bottle A, Clark SK, Darzi AW, Aylin P. Elective colonic surgery for cancer in the elderly: an investigation into postoperative mortality in English NHS hospitals between 1996 and 2007. Colorectal Dis. 2011;13(7):779–85.

22. Audisio RA, Pope D, Ramesh HS, Gennari R, van Leeuwen BL, West C, et al. Shall we operate? Preoperative assessment in elderly cancer patients (PACE) can help. A SIOG surgical task force prospective study. Crit Rev Oncol Hematol. 2008;65(2):156–63.

23. Kristjansson SR, Nesbakken A, Jordhoy MS, Skovlund E, Audisio RA, Johannessen HO, et al. Comprehensive geriatric assessment can predict complications in elderly patients after elective surgery for colorectal cancer: a prospective observational cohort study. Crit Rev Oncol Hematol. 2010;76(3):208–17.

24. Sunouchi K, Namiki K, Mori M, Shimizu T, Tadokoro M. How should patients 80 years of age or older with colorectal carcinoma be treated? Long-term and short-term outcome and postoperative cytokine levels. Dis Colon Rectum. 2000;43(2):233–41.

25. Gurevitch AJ, Davidovitch B, Kashtan H. Outcome of right colectomy for cancer in octogenarians. J Gastrointest Surg. 2009;13(1):100–4.

26. Kehlet H. Fast-track colorectal surgery. Lancet. 2008;371(9615):791–3.

27. de Vries EN, Prins HA, Crolla RM, den Outer AJ, van Andel G, van Helden SH, et al. Effect of a comprehensive surgical safety system on patient outcomes. N Engl J Med. 2010;363(20): 1928–37.

28. Law WL, Chu KW, Tung PH. Laparoscopic colorectal resection: a safe option for elderly patients. J Am Coll Surg. 2002;195(6):768–73.
29. Kristjansson SR, Jordhøy MS, Nesbakken A, Skovlund E, Bakka A, Johannessen H, et al. Which elements of a comprehensive geriatric assessment (CGA) predict post-operative complications and early mortality after colorectal cancer surgery? J Geriatr Oncol. 2010;1(2): 57–65.

Chapter 5
Comprehensive Geriatric Assessment

Margot A. Gosney and Priya Das

Abstract We live within an ageing population, and those over the age of 85 years will continue to make up increasing numbers and overall total proportion of populations across the world. In the UK, the number of older people aged 85 years and above will more than double in the next 25 years. In 2034, it is predicted that over 3.5 million of the UK population will be aged 85 years or above. This coupled with increasing numbers of older people developing colorectal cancer will result in large numbers of this population presenting to the hospital, either as emergencies or elective admissions for the management of their cancer. While some cancers can be diagnosed and treated in the outpatient setting, a number of tumor types require admission for surgery and for more prolonged chemotherapy and radiotherapy. This is the case in colorectal cancer (CRC). Older patients are at higher risk of adverse effects, including long inpatient stays, increased complications, higher readmission rates, and increased rates of placement in long-term care facilities. In nearly every setting where older people are cared for, a comprehensive geriatric assessment (CGA) is performed. The CGA is defined as "a multi-dimensional, inter disciplinary diagnostic process to determine the medical, psychological and functional capabilities of a frail older person, in order to develop a co-ordinated, integrated plan for treatment and long term follow up." In general geriatric medicine, CGA is considered to be the gold standard when caring for older people in hospital. There are, however, a number of issues which have not been fully evaluated. These include the following.

Keywords CGA • Comprehensive geriatric assessment • Frailty • Geriatric assessment • Cancer surgery • Elderly • Colorectal cancer

M.A. Gosney, M.D., FRCP(✉)
Elderly Care Medicine, University of Reading/Royal Berkshire NHS Foundation Trust,
London Road, Reading, Berkshire RG1 5AQ, UK
e-mail: m.a.gosney@reading.ac.uk

P. Das, MBBS
Royal Berkshire NHS Foundation Trust,
London Road, Reading, UK

D. Papamichael, R.A. Audisio (eds.), *Management of Colorectal Cancers in Older People*,
DOI 10.1007/978-0-85729-984-0_5, © Springer-Verlag London 2013

Introduction

We live within an ageing population, and those over the age of 85 years will continue to make up increasing numbers and overall total proportion of populations across the world. In the UK, the number of older people aged 85 years and above will more than double in the next 25 years. In 2034, it is predicted that over 3.5 million of the UK population will be aged 85 years or above. This coupled with increasing numbers of older people developing colorectal cancer will result in large numbers of this population presenting to the hospital, either as emergencies or elective admissions for the management of their cancer. While some cancers can be diagnosed and treated in the outpatient setting, a number of tumor types require admission for surgery and for more prolonged chemotherapy and radiotherapy. This is the case in colorectal cancer (CRC). Older patients are at higher risk of adverse effects, including long inpatient stays, increased complications, higher readmission rates, and increased rates of placement in long-term care facilities. In nearly every setting where older people are cared for, a comprehensive geriatric assessment (CGA) is performed. The CGA is defined as "a multi-dimensional, inter disciplinary diagnostic process to determine the medical, psychological and functional capabilities of a frail older person, in order to develop a co-ordinated, integrated plan for treatment and long term follow up." In general geriatric medicine, CGA is considered to be the gold standard when caring for older people in hospital. There are, however, a number of issues which have not been fully evaluated. These include the following.

Why Do We Need to Assess Older People with Cancer?

Following diagnosis, the comprehensive geriatric assessment (CGA) is a tool used alongside the general and colorectal cancer-specific examinations. It examines factors affecting the elderly patient, namely, the medical comorbidities, and any functional, social, or psychological limitations [1]. Its role is well recognized in the management of the elderly cancer patient [2–7], and it allows more efficient care of elderly patients than other scales [8, 9].

Since age cannot predict outcome in an elderly cancer patient, the CGA aids management by helping to identify those who will benefit from curative treatment and those who will be best treated with palliation. The tool can also monitor progress of a patient while they receive treatment as CGA can be conducted before, during, and after therapy.

CGA has demonstrated that large amounts of comorbidity exist alongside the diagnosed cancer and that this also impacts on a cancer patient's functional state. In 2001, Serraino and colleagues looked at 300 patients above 65 years with cancer. They showed that poor performance status independently affected both ADL (activities of daily living) and IADL (instrumental activities of daily living) disability. Furthermore, 17 % had limitations in ADL and 59 % for IADLs [10]. Within the last

20 years, there has been an increasing awareness that geriatric oncology is a specialty in its own right. More recently, there has been an understanding of the role of comorbidity and that not only diagnosing comorbidity but also optimizing clinical status improves the management of patients with cancer. The giants of geriatric medicine, as described by Bernard Isaacs (incontinence, instability, and falls; impaired hearing and vision; and intellectual decline), have an increasing prevalence with every decade of increasing age.

Is the Same CGA Required in CRC as in General Geriatric Practice?

The comprehensive geriatric assessment, if used correctly, evaluates a number of aspects of what are considered to be normal ageing. Due to the areas that it covers, it enables patients to be thoroughly assessed in a holistic fashion, and therefore, comorbidities identified can be treated prior to embarking on definitive treatment for the newly diagnosed condition. While there is no gold standard as to what CGA comprises, the components in Table 5.1 are felt to be integral to the assessment process.

In a 2011 study by Buurman, patients over the age of 65 years who were admitted acutely to hospital for at least 2 days were assessed with regard to their comorbidity. While 83 % of them had IADL impairment, 61 % polypharmacy, 59 % mobility difficulty, and over half had high levels of primary caregiver burden and malnutrition, these were not fully reported in discharge summaries. Only the presence of polypharmacy and cognitive impairment were likely to be highlighted. Just 12 months after admission, 35 % of these individuals had died and 33 % suffered from functional decline. A poor outcome was predicted by a high Charlson comorbidity index score, the presence of malnutrition, high falls risk, and presence of delirium, as well as premorbid IADL impairment [11]. Not only does this paper identify high levels of comorbidity and geriatric syndromes but also indicates that

Table 5.1 Components integral to the assessment process

Component	Element
Medical assessment	Colorectal cancer stage (including measures needed for symptom control)
	Comorbidities (and need for optimization)
	Medication review (including polypharmacy)
	Nutritional state
	Diagnosis of asymptomatic conditions
Psychological state	Mini mental state examination
	Depression screening
Social assessment	Formal and informal care requirements
Functional status	Activities of daily living (as well as instrumental ADLs)
	Activity/exercise status
	Gait and balance

early detection does not always occur, documentation on discharge to enable primary caregivers to optimize patients is often lacking, and all of these measures of impairment are indicative of poor outcome. The evidence of the effectiveness of CGA in the care of older people in a variety of settings was identified in a number of randomized controlled trials reported by Ferrucci et al. in 2003 [12].

Although some of the earlier systematic reviews have identified large numbers of trials where CGA has been employed (28 trials), many of the older studies have looked at geriatric medicine services, such as day hospital and hospital at home, and therefore, delivery of CGA in some settings which are now considered to be inefficient may have impacted upon the overall efficacy of the CGA [13]. In studies of older patients in the emergency department where initial CGA and follow-up at home for 28 days was compared with usual care, researchers found lower levels of readmission during the first 38 days (16.5 % vs. 22.2 % $P=0.048$), lower rate of emergency admissions during an 18-month follow-up period (44.4 % vs. 54.3 % $P=0.007$), and a longer time to first emergency admission (382 vs. 348 days, $P=0.011$) in the CGA group. The finding of improved physical function, as measured by the Barthel index at 6 months, is not surprising in the intervention group; however, cognitive function also seems to improve, which requires further explanation.

The evidence for the usefulness of CGA has been identified in a number of studies. A systematic review undertaken in 2008 showed that older people admitted to conventional care units had a worse outcome than those who were admitted to acute geriatric medicine units where a comprehensive geriatric assessment was undertaken. Those who had CGA performed had a lower risk of functional decline at discharge and were more likely to live at home after discharge. There was no difference, however, in case fatality, and the meta-analysis included 11 studies, of which 5 were randomized trials, 4 nonrandomized trials, and 2 were case-controlled studies [14]. Similar studies analyzing the effect of home visitations with comprehensive geriatric assessment in order to prevent nursing home admission and functional decline have shown similar findings with over 13,000 individuals being included within the analysis [15, 16].

With increasing pressures, both financial and on total bed numbers, it is important that comprehensive geriatric assessment reduces length of stay, without impacting on patient outcomes. This has been particularly well studied in the USA, where centralization of funding and accurate cost recording have shown that length of stay for inpatient rehabilitation substantially decreased from 1994 to 2001, while functional status changes have maintained constant and discharge destination has not deteriorated [17]. The role of comprehensive geriatric assessment within rehabilitation to accurately target input also highlights the need to ensure the cost-effectiveness is considered, as well as quality of life and quality-adjusted life-year scoring. The increasing emphasis on care delivered in the community makes comprehensive geriatric assessment at the time of presentation even more important. While in some settings the care of older people in community hospitals is considered to be less expensive than in a tertiary center, this is not a consistent finding, which once again stresses the need for CGA to be undertaken and then rapidly acted upon, with resultant early discharge home to the community, not into either a general or rehabilitation hospital, if this can be avoided [18].

It must be increasingly stressed that the undertaking of a CGA will not improve outcomes without focused action, often over a prolonged period. Conroy et al. in 2011 identified studies of older people who were discharged home within 72 h after they had been assessed with a comprehensive geriatric assessment. They found no clear evidence of benefit from CGA interventions in this population in terms of mortality, readmissions, subsequent institutionalization, functional ability, quality of life, or cognition [19]. This population if fit for such quick discharge will probably be more fit than those undergoing treatment for CRC in whom CGA is being considered.

Should All Patients Over the Age of 70 Years with Cancer Undergo CGA?

At the beginning of this century, there were some doubts as to which patients should undergo CGA [20]. While older, more frail patients with cancer should undergo CGA, it has become clearer in the last 10–15 years that even fit, older cancer patients may benefit from such a comprehensive assessment.

We have a greater understanding of frailty, and this is increasingly being applied to older oncology patients. While some authors have defined frailty and then used a comprehensive geriatric assessment in order to reverse those factors that are reversible, there are others who have constructed and validated frailty indices, basing them on routinely used comprehensive geriatric assessment instruments [21]. The review by Ferrucci highlights the evolution of the CGA and its use in older cancer patients. While many of the early papers suggest a brief but standard CGA protocol, this has evolved to focus more on comorbidity associated with cancer [22]. There appears to be adequate evidence to justify the design and conduct of randomized controlled trials to test the effectiveness of CGA in the care, management, and follow-up of cancer patients, although this has only occurred in a piecemeal, unstandardized, and anecdotal nature. There is the suggestion that the current CGA instruments are more useful in the assessment of older patients who are sick and disabled than to assess instability of health or susceptibility to side effects or complications in those who are elderly but fit. This may reflect different CGA protocols but also whether the CGA is merely used as a diagnostic, rather than a diagnostic and therapeutic aid. It is important to highlight that some of the performance status instruments used in everyday life, such as the Karnofsky Performance Status Scale, was first published in 1968 [23]. Likewise, other geriatric medicine scales such as the Barthel index are over 50 years since their original inception [24]. Unfortunately, the Karnofsky score lacks sensitivity and specificity, but the Barthel score remains a good measure of basic activities of daily living and is still incorporated in most CGA protocols.

Frailty predicts hospitalization and visits to primary care physicians and also to emergency departments in newly diagnosed cancer patients [25] including those with colorectal cancer. While this chapter found that those elderly individuals with one or more markers of frailty were frequently encountered, it was only cognitive impairment that predicted emergency department visits. While this highlights the prevalence of frailty, it also goes some way toward explaining why some older individuals with colorectal cancer may underutilize healthcare services unless people have proactively sought out comorbidity and the giants of geriatric medicine [25].

What Are We Trying to Evaluate with the CGA?

The main reason for a CGA is that age-related changes occur at different rates in different individuals and do not reflect chronological age. The geriatric oncology task force (EORTC), whose aim is to improve the management of older cancer patients, has suggested a two-step approach. This focus is on an early screening either in the community or the hospital, performed by an oncologist or the geriatrician, determining whether the patient is fit or frail. Those fit patients then undergo usual care with the oncologist providing all the necessary coordination. Those who are identified as frail are combined with those from long-term care facilities and have a geriatrician-led CGA, which results in either geriatric palliative care or an interdisciplinary team determining a modified approach to that individual's cancer management [26, 27]. Certain areas within the CGA are of particular importance in colorectal cancer. It is known that nutritional status independently predicts disability and mortality in older patients [28]. Tolerance to antineoplastic treatments and delayed recovery of normal tissue after chemotherapy is entirely predictable by nutritional status. Prolonged fasting prior to the diagnosis of colorectal cancer during CT or endoscopy does little to improve the nutritional status of older individuals when they first present to the oncologist. Postoperative nausea, ileus, and impaired mobility also diminish calorie intake. Poor nutrition is often combined with cognitive impairment and puts this group at increased risk. The EORTC position paper on the approach to the older cancer patient highlighted the role of geriatric assessment in the selection of elderly cancer patients who were suitable for definitive treatment [29]. It must also be remembered that CGA, as well as providing a global view on the patient, may in the future be used as a tool for stratifying and/or randomizing patients in clinical studies [29].

Should the CGA Be a Two-Step Process, with an Abbreviated Form Identifying Those Who Will Benefit Most from a More Detailed Version?

Two papers, published in 2005 and 2006, by Obercash and colleagues, identified that an abbreviated CGA could be helpful in screening those older individuals who benefit from the entire CGA [30, 31]. They used a 15-item abbreviated CGA and found that the Cronbach's alpha was 0.65–0.92 on each instrument of the entire CGA, compared to 0.70–0.94 on the abbreviated CGA. They suggested that a low score in the abbreviated CGA in any of the four domains (functional status, instrumental activities of daily living, depression, and cognition) would result in a more focused CGA being undertaken. However, a low score in one domain should not necessarily result in all four domains being studied intensively. The study included 500 retrospectively reviewed charts of patients, of whom 12 % had a primary diagnosis of colon cancer. The abbreviated CGA took an undetermined amount of time, and it is difficult to tell from these retrospective studies how much intervention occurred after the initial abbreviated CGA.

Can the CGA Be Used to Determine Which Patients Are Most Suited for Which Treatments, Those Patients Who Are Most Likely to Undergo Significant Morbidity During Treatment, and Can It Be Used as a Predictor of Long-Term Outcome?

While we have presented evidence that the routine use of CGA has a positive effect on health outcomes, it is important to determine at which time during the cancer journey the CGA is most effective. CGA must be used to evaluate all aspects of ageing so that the care plan can be tailored to the patient. It should help determine those individuals who are candidates for standard treatment to prolong life, as well as those in whom the potential benefits of such treatment are outweighed by its risks. While the latter group may not benefit from definitive treatment of their cancer, they may still benefit from modified regimens with a palliative intent or even due to the medical management of outstanding preexisting conditions, irrespective of the underlying cancer.

Prior to undertaking a decision about definitive treatment, the CGA will help to identify the life expectancy of an individual patient. CGA should be used to detect important conditions that are associated with short survival, and this is mainly assessed through performance status, ability to perform ADLs, and the presence or absence of comorbidity [32, 33]. Life expectancy is also dependent on frailty, and the 2-year mortality rate is much higher in long-term recipients of institutional care than in those who are fully independent (40 % vs. 8 %) [34].

The next consideration is whether older patients with colorectal cancer are able to tolerate surgery, chemotherapy, and radiotherapy. One of the major factors to consider in all three modalities is the presence of malnutrition. Guigoz and colleagues identified the high prevalence of malnutrition in older hospitalized or institutionalized individuals [35]. If impaired nutrition is not reversed, poor wound healing and pressure area instability following surgery, as well as increased toxic effects of chemotherapy due to low protein binding, are particular hazards in this patient group.

Discharge planning and response to rehabilitation are affected by depression due to its role in motivation for treatment [36]. Therefore, depression and anxiety are as important as cognition in the CGA assessment.

Should the CGA Be Administered in Hospital or in the Community Setting?

It is essential that CGA is initially undertaken when the patient first presents. While the majority of studies have administered the CGA in hospital, it is our finding that over 75 % patients wish their initial assessment to be undertaken in their own home (data on request from authors). While this is clearly more time-consuming, it does enable some aspects of patient assessment to be undertaken without the recourse to other healthcare professionals. The patient can be assessed in their own environment, and this is a way of validating some of the statements made by patients who may be falsely suggesting that their social situation is better than it is truly and in those with mild cognitive impairment who may not accurately report home circumstances. We have found that assessment of bed and chair height, adequacy of bathing and kitchen facilities, and access to and from buildings, as well as the opportunity to meet with other family members and primary healthcare providers in the patient's own home, is worth the additional time burden. In a report by Extermann, when CGA was undertaken in patients with early breast cancer, a 3-monthly assessment by a multidisciplinary team, as well as a monthly telephone call, resulted in large numbers of unaddressed or under-addressed problems at the initial examination, as well as an average of three new problems over the following 6 months [37]. This, however, has not been replicated in CRC. In some studies, it is a primary nurse practitioner who administers the core geriatric assessment with the input of a dietician, a social worker, and a pharmacist. This allows the case to be summarized and presented to the oncologist, who then meets the patient with a thorough understanding of their other issues [38]. In other models, after initial screening, a patient may be seen by a geriatrician in consultation in the clinic. However, if the screening suggests a large number of issues, the patient is referred to the geriatric department for a complete evaluation. This may result in "at-risk patients" receiving a comprehensive geriatric assessment by the geriatricians but with an added delay in the start of definitive treatment for their cancer.

Can Models of Care That Have Been Identified as Cost-Effective Using CGA Be Readily Transferred to Other Areas of Cancer Care?

As already discussed under "Who should undertake the CGA?," there is evidence that a geriatrician who is skilled at diagnosis and management of a variety of underlying geriatric syndromes should be involved in the care of the older patient with cancer. There are predictors of greater lengths of stay in older patients admitted to hospital. These include falls, development of delirium, uncontrolled pain, and urinary incontinence. The use of an older person's assessment and liaison team to deliver CGA through a multidisciplinary team including a nurse, physiotherapist, and geriatrician results in reduced length of stay and overall improved clinical effectiveness and hospital performance [39]. Such a multidisciplinary team has not been studied in the cancer setting, although the combination of nurse and doctor has been highlighted in the Department of Health and Macmillan pilot sites in the United Kingdom [38]. The extension of multidisciplinary preoperative CGA, combined with postoperative follow-through, is pertinent to the surgical management of colorectal cancer. In elective orthopedic patient, such an intervention reduces postoperative complications, including pneumonia (20 % vs. 4 % $P=0.008$) and delirium (19 % vs. 6 % $P=0.036$), and results in significant improvement in areas such as pressure area management, pain control, delayed mobilization, and inappropriate catheter use, reflecting the element of multidisciplinary input. Overall, the length of stay was also reduced by 4.5 days. While this study was in elective surgical patients who had undergone orthopedic procedures, one can see how this might relate to colorectal surgery [40].

In order for CGA to involve geriatricians, there needs to be an understanding of the needs of the oncology patient by the geriatrician. In 2010, Puts and colleagues undertook a qualitative study of physicians from the Department of Oncology and the Division of Medicine. Twenty-four cancer specialists and 17 geriatricians agreed to participate using semi-structured interviews and a topic guide, asking similar questions to both groups of clinicians. Overall, the majority of oncologists had developed their own form of assessment of older people with cancer, which consisted primarily of functional status and some information on comorbidity. The only specific tools that they reported were the European Cooperative Oncology Group performance status (ECOG) and the Karnofsky scale for function. On the other hand, geriatricians used structured comprehensive geriatric assessment for their older patients. Of interest, half of the cancer specialists indicated that their patients did not need a referral to a geriatrician but they would refer as it was required. The geriatricians stress that the cancer specialists predominantly referred patients for geriatric syndromes, such as falls, delirium, fractures, or cognitive impairment, not specifically because they were an older person with cancer. While cancer specialists wanted more support systems to be available and more access to social workers and psychologists, they also stated that transportation services needed to improve, as well as better collaboration with the GP. In contrast, the geriatricians unanimously felt that they needed better communication between geriatricians and cancer specialists. While both groups of clinicians wanted further exploration of quality of life issues, the geriatricians were keen to study whether CGA predicted the outcome of cancer and its treatment [41].

The French National Cancer Institute created pilot oncogeriatric coordination units to implement routine geriatric assessment of all cancer patients over 75 years of age. While these pilot units were to target problems such as late diagnosis, late management, incomplete investigations, and poorer prognosis due to less intensive treatment than in younger populations, it draws an ideal population and collaborative system to study the role of the status of the geriatrician in the management of older patients with cancer [42]. While cancer specialists on the whole started to perceive the geriatricians intervention as a means to improve the management of elderly cancer patients, they wanted it to occur only in situations in which they considered it necessary. Cancer specialists considered it undermined their independence in decision-making, particularly around the age criteria. There was, however, evidence that cancer specialists did use the geriatricians expertise, before and after multidisciplinary consultation meetings. Since most countries now have an obligatory multidisciplinary team meeting for therapeutic decision-making, this provides evidence that the geriatricians involvement should be both before and after such meetings. It is important therefore, in the use of comprehensive geriatric assessment, that geriatricians do not become excluded from the process. Efficacy will be reduced if they do not have a coherent role, in other words, one that is not dependent on upstream decisions by cancer specialists, which results in their intervention being too late or in a random matter. In addition, geriatricians need to feel valued to ensure that they do not become merely a handmaiden of the cancer team [43].

There is little doubt that older age influences cancer management. Comorbidity, frailty, and the giants of geriatric medicine make surgeons and oncologists nervous about undertaking rigorous and potentially life-limiting therapy. Even with the non-geriatricians, those working day to day with older people may not be fully aware of their ageist attitudes. Foster et al. studied 200 oncologists via an e-mail study, to determine their behavior in the management of older individuals. All oncologists were seeing at least 20 patients per week, of whom 10 % were patients aged over 65 years [43]. When considering a woman with metastatic colon cancer for whom chemotherapy was recommended, nearly all oncologists chose an intensive regime if the patient's age was 63, but if her age was 85, approximately 25 % of oncologists would choose a less intensive treatment. No oncologist would suggest single-agent chemotherapy alone for the 63-year-old, but 80 % chose this option for the 85-year-old. Combination chemotherapy followed by surgery was recommended for 31.6 % of the 63-year-olds but only 18.6 % of the 85-year-olds. All comparisons reached statistical significance, $P=0.001$.

We are also fully aware that while the UK has a lower burden of chronic conditions, there are still approximately 15.4 million people in England with long-term conditions, of whom 60 % are aged over 60 years. Within the next 25 years, this will rise by nearly a quarter, and the most common condition is arthritis, which accounts for almost 28 % of all long-term conditions. The impact of arthritis on a patient with colorectal cancer may be through impaired mobility, manual dexterity to deal with stoma, or late diagnosis of bowel cancer due to change in bowel habit, being attributed to medication for underlying orthopedic conditions [44]. It is also known that the major rise in psychological conditions will be in dementia. Many individuals with mild cognitive impairment through to advanced dementia will have a diagnosis of colorectal cancer. Delirium will be an increasing postoperative complication, and the management of postoperative pain will be ladened with difficulties. To ensure the development of the comprehensive geriatric assessment will keep abreast of changing patient groups, new methodologies need to be employed [45].

What Is the Evidence for CGA in Colorectal Cancer?

The clinical assessment of elderly people with cancer has been studied and published in a number of reviews [46]. However, there is a poverty of data that specifically reviews the role of CGA in colorectal cancer. With regard to comprehensive geriatric assessment and postoperative complications, a prospective study of 178 consecutive patients over 70 years who had elective surgery for colorectal cancer was examined. The preoperative CGA was used to categorize patients as fit, intermediate, or frail. This was combined with an outcome measure of severe complications within 30 days of surgery. Not surprisingly, approximately half of the patients were characterized as intermediate (46 %), with 43 % as frail and only 12 % categorized as fit. Severe complications occurred in 33 % of fit, 36 % of intermediate, and 62 % of frail patients. Age and ASA classification were not associated with risk of complications [47]. Unfortunately, however, this does little to help determine which aspect of the CGA predicted the outcome and, indeed, which abnormalities within the CGA were potentially reversible and what effects this would have had on outcome after colorectal cancer surgery.

Even more recently, published papers looking at novel approaches to perioperative assessment and intervention do little to explore the specific gaps in understanding longitudinal patient-centered outcomes of colorectal cancer treatment and how this might be affected by CGA. Cheema and colleagues suggest that short-term rather than long-term complications can be predicted by CGA, although this has not been a universal finding in other tumor types [48]. While some authors have suggested that CGA may help age treatment decisions around the administration of chemotherapy for colorectal cancer, it is difficult to validate the reduction of duration of treatment or intensity of treatment in frail, older patients without a thorough evaluation through a randomized controlled trial. While there has been little in the way of trials specifically in older people with colorectal cancer undergoing chemotherapy, similar trials in breast cancer have been terminated early due to poor recruitment [49, 50]. What is known, however, is that relatively fit, elderly patients with a variety of advanced tumors, including colorectal cancer, can have palliative benefit from treatment but with predictable toxicity when coexisting conditions such as low serum albumen and renal dysfunction are identified [51].

Summary

Colorectal cancer will continue to be a challenge in older people and, with increasing age, will cover a larger proportion of increasingly frail individuals. Comprehensive geriatric assessment is well validated in older patients, and indeed, there is increasing evidence of its usefulness in older patients with cancer. However, doubt still remains as to whether CGA can be used to stratify treatment decisions and to entirely predict surgical and oncological complications. Where doubt has been eradicated is in the knowledge that CGA, without intervention, is at best useless and, at worst, ageist and unethical. The delivery of CGA in whatever format should be by a multidisciplinary team, which includes a geriatrician. Patient selection must not be determined by the oncologist but by robust screening methodologies. Increasing collaboration between the geriatrician and those caring for oncology patients is essential to ensure that resources are correctly targeted and patients benefit, both in terms of longevity and quality of life.

References

1. Monfardini S, Balducci L. A comprehensive geriatric assessment is necessary for study and the management of cancer in the elderly. Eur J Cancer. 1999;35:1771–2.
2. Repetto L, Granetto C, Venturino A. Comorbidity and cancer in the aged: the oncologists point of view. Rays. 1997;22:17–9.
3. Repetto L, Comandini D. Cancer in the elderly: assessing patients for fitness. Crit Rev Oncol Hematol. 2000;35:155–60.
4. Repetto L, Ausili-Cefaro G, Gallo C, Rossi A, Manzione L. Quality of life in elderly cancer patients. Ann Oncol. 2001;12:S49–52.
5. Repetto L, Fratino L, Audisio RA, et al. Comprehensive geriatric assessment adds information to Eastern Cooperative Oncology Group Performance status in elderly care patients: an Italian Group for Geriatric Oncology Study. J Clin Oncol. 2002;20:494–502.
6. Wells JL, Seabrook JA, Stolee P, Borrie MJ, Knoefel F. State of the art in geriatric rehabilitation. Part I: review of frailty and comprehensive geriatric assessment. Arch Phys Med Rehabil. 2003;84(6):890–7.
7. Baztan JJ, Suarez Garcia FM, Lopez-Arrieta J, Rodriguez-Manas L, Rodriguez-Artalejo F. Effectiveness of acute geriatric units on functional decline, living at home, and case fatality among older patients admitted to hospital for acute medical disorders: meta-analysis. BMJ. 2009;338:b50.
8. Bernabei R, Venturiero V, Tarsitani P, Gambassi G. The comprehensive geriatric assessment: when, where, how. Crit Rev Oncol Hematol. 2000;33:45–6.
9. Repetto L, Venturino A, Fratino L, et al. Geriatric oncology: a clinical approach to the older patient with cancer. Eur J Cancer. 2003;39:870–80.
10. Serraino D, Fratino L, Zagonel V, GIOGer Study Group (Italy). Prevalence of functional disability among elderly patients with cancer. Crit Rev Oncol Hematol. 2001;39:269–73.
11. Buurman BM, Hoogerduijn JG, De Haan RJ, Abu-Hanna A, et al. Geriatric conditions in acutely hospitalized older patients: prevalence and one-year survival and functional decline. PLoS One. 2011;6:e26951.
12. Ferrucci L, Guralnik JM, Cavazzini C, Bandinelli S, Lauretani F, Bartali B, et al. The frailty syndrome: a critical issue in geriatric oncology. Crit Rev Oncol Hematol. 2003; 46(2):127–37.
13. Stuck AE, Siu AL, Wieland GD, Adams J, Rubenstein LZ. Comprehensive geriatric assessment: a meta-analysis of controlled trials. Lancet. 1993;342(8878):1032–6.
14. Baztán JJ, Suárez-García FM, López-Arrieta J, et al. Effectiveness of acute geriatric units on functional decline, living at home, and case fatality among older patients admitted to hospital for acute medical disorders: meta-analysis. BMJ. 2009;338:b50.
15. Stuck AE, Egger M, Hammer A, et al. Home visits to prevent nursing home admission and functional decline in elderly people. Systematic review and meta-regression analysis. JAMA. 2002;287:1022–8.

16. Bachmann S, Finger C, Huss A, et al. Inpatient rehabilitation specifically designed for geriatric patients: systematic review and meta-analysis of randomised controlled trials. BMJ. 2010;340:c1718.
17. Ottenbacher KJ, Smith PM, Illig SB, et al. Trends in length of stay, living setting, functional outcome, and mortality following medical rehabilitation. JAMA. 2004;292:1687–95.
18. O'Reilly J, Lowson K, Green J, et al. Post-acute care for older people in community hospitals – a cost-effectiveness analysis within a multi-centre randomised controlled trial. Age Ageing. 2008;37:513–20.
19. Conroy SP, Stevens T, Parker SG, Gladman JRF. A systematic review of comprehensive geriatric assessment to improve outcomes for frail older people being rapidly discharged from acute hospital: 'interface geriatrics'. Age Ageing. 2011;40:436–43.
20. Extermann M, Aapro M, Bernabei R, et al. Use of comprehensive geriatric assessment in older cancer patients: recommendations from the task force on CGA of the International Society of Geriatric Oncology (SIOG). Crit Rev Oncol Hematol. 2005;3:241–52.
21. Jones DM, Song X, Rockwood K. Operationalizing a frailty index from a standardized comprehensive geriatric assessment. J Am Geriatr Soc. 2004;52:1929–33.
22. Ferrucci L, Guralnik JM, Cavazzini C, Bandinelli S, et al. The frailty syndrome: a critical issue in geriatric oncology. Crit Rev Oncol Hematol. 2003;46:127–37.
23. Karnofsky DA. Determining the extent of the cancer and clinical planning for cure. Cancer. 1968;22:730–4.
24. Barthel DW, Mahoney FI. Functional evaluation: the Barthel Index. Md State Med J. 1965;14:61–5.
25. Puts MTE, Monette J, Girre V, Wolfson C, et al. Does frailty predict hospitalization, emergency department visits, and visits to the general practitioner in older newly-diagnosed cancer patients? Results of a prospective pilot study. Crit Rev Oncol Hematol. 2010;76:142–51.
26. Balducci L, Colloca G, Cesari M, Gambassi G. Assessment and treatment of elderly patients with cancer. Surg Oncol. 2010;19:117–23.
27. Extermann M, Aapro M, Bernabei R, et al. Use of comprehensive geriatric assessment in older cancer patients: recommendations from the task force on CGA of the international society of geriatric oncology (SIOG). Crit Rev Oncol Hematol. 2005;55:241–2.
28. Sharkey JR. The interrelationship of nutritional risk factors, indicators of nutritional risk, and severity of disability among home-delivered meal participants. Gerontologist. 2002;42:373–80.
29. Pallis AG, Fortpied C, Wedding U, Van Nes MC, et al. EORTC elderly task force position paper: approach to the older cancer patient. Eur J Cancer. 2010;46:1502–13.
30. Overcash JA, Beckstead J, Extermann M, Cobb S. The abbreviated comprehensive geriatric assessment (aCGA): a retrospective analysis. Crit Rev Oncol Hematol. 2005;54:129–36.
31. Overcash JA, Beckstead J, Moody L, Extermann M, Cobb S. The abbreviated comprehensive geriatric assessment (aCGA) for use in the older cancer patient as a prescreen: scoring and interpretation. Crit Rev Oncol Hematol. 2006;59:205–10.
32. Reuben DB, Rubenstein LV, Hirsch SH, et al. Value of functional status as a predictor of mortality: results for a prospective study. Medicine. 1992;6:663–9.
33. Yancik R, Wesley MN, Ries LAG, et al. Comorbidity and age as predictors of risk for early mortality of male and female colon carcinoma patients: a population-based study. Cancer. 1998;82(11): 2123–34.
34. Balducci L, Stanta S. Cancer in the frail patient: a coming epidemic. Hematol Oncol Clin North Am. 2000;14:235–50.
35. Guigoz Y, Lauque S, Vellas BJ. Identifying the elderly at risk for malnutrition. The mini nutritional assessment. Clin Geriatr Med. 2002;18:737–57.
36. Balducci L. New paradigms for treating elderly patients with cancer: the comprehensive geriatric assessment and guidelines for supportive care. J Support Oncol. 2003;1:30–7.
37. Extermann M. Studies of comprehensive geriatric assessment in patients with cancer. Cancer Control. 2003;10:463–8.

38. http://www.macmillan.org.uk/Aboutus/Healthprofessionals/Improvingservicesforolderpeople/Pilots/PilotsiteThamesValley.aspx. Accessed on Sept. 9, 2012.

39. Harari D, Martin FC, Buttery A, et al. The older persons' assessment and liaison team 'OPAL': evaluation of comprehensive and geriatric assessment in acute medical inpatients. Age Ageing. 2007;36:670–5.

40. Harari D, Hopper A, Jugdeep D, et al. Proactive care for older people undergoing surgery ('POPS'): designing, embedding, evaluating and funding a comprehensive geriatric assessment service for older elective surgical patients. Age Ageing. 2007;36:190–6.

41. Puts MTE, Girre V, Wolfson C, et al. Clinical experience of cancer specialists and geriatricians involved in cancer care of older patients: a qualitative study. Crit Rev Oncol Hematol. 2010;74:87–96.

42. Sifer-Riviere L, Saint-Jeab O, Gisselbrecht M, et al. What the specific tools of geriatrics and oncology can tell us about the role and status of geriatricians in a pilot geriatric oncology program. Ann Oncol. 2011;22:2325–9.

43. Foster JA, Salinas GD, Mansell SD, et al. How does older age influence oncologists' cancer management? Oncologist. 2010;15:584–92.

44. Berzins K, Reilly S, Abell J, et al. UK self-care support initiatives for older patients with long-term conditions: a review. Chronic Illn. 2009;5:56–72.

45. Zwakhalen SMG, Hamers JPH, Berger MPF. The psychometric quality and clinical usefulness of three pain assessment tools for elderly people with dementia. Pain. 2006;126:210–20.

46. Gosney MA. Clinical assessment of elderly people with cancer. Lancet Oncol. 2005;6:790–7.

47. Kristjansson SR, Nesbakken A, et al. Comprehensive geriatric assessment can predict complications in elderly patients after elective surgery for colorectal cancer: a prospective observational cohort study. Crit Rev Oncol Hematol. 2010;76:208–17.

48. Cheema FN, Abraham NS, Berger DH, et al. Novel approaches to perioperative assessment and intervention may improve long-term outcomes after colorectal cancer resection in older adults. Ann Surg. 2011;253:867–74.

49. Droz JP, Aapro M, Balducci L. Overcoming challenges associated with chemotherapy treatment in the senior adult population. Crit Rev Oncol Hematol. 2008;68 Suppl 1:S1–8.

50. Leonard R, Ballinger R, Cameron D, et al. Adjuvant chemotherapy in older women (ACTION) study – what did we learn from the pilot phase? Br J Cancer. 2011;25:1260–6.

51. Pentheroudakis G, Fiuntzilas G, Kalofonos HP. Palliative chemotherapy in elderly patients with common metastatic malignancies: a Hellenic Cooperative Oncology Group registry analysis of management, outcome and clinical benefit predictors. Crit Rev Oncol Hematol. 2008;66:237–47.

Chapter 6
Surgical Treatment of Colorectal Cancer in Older Patients

Harm J.T. Rutten, Gerrit-Jan Liefers, and Valery E.P. P. Lemmens

Abstract Elderly colorectal cancer patients are underrepresented in randomized studies. Despite the fact that modern guidelines are evidence based, they may not be considered validated for the compromised elderly patient. Increasing age and comorbidity decrease the physiological reserves to respond adequately to occurring complications. Acute surgery also is a major challenge for the older colorectal cancer patient. As a result, before counseling an older patient with colon or rectal cancer, a thorough somatic and mental assessment has to be performed in order to give the best treatment advice, considering primarily the patient's and his or her family's perspective.

Keywords Elderly • Colorectal cancer • Rectal cancer • Surgery • Frailty • Aged • Complications • Assessment • Counseling

H.J.T. Rutten, M.D., Ph.D., FRCS (London) (✉)
Colorectal Surgery, Catharina Hospital Eindhoven,
Michelangelolaan 2, Eindhoven, Noord Brabant 5623 EJ, The Netherlands
e-mail: hrutten@xs4all.nl

G.-J. Liefers, M.D., Ph.D.
Department of Surgery, Leiden University Medical Center,
Albinusdreef 2, Leiden 2333 ZA, The Netherlands

V.E.P.P. Lemmens, Ph.D.
Department of Research, Comprehensive Cancer Centre South,
Zernikestraat 29, P.O. Box 231, Eindhoven 2600 AE, The Netherlands

Department of Public Health, Erasmus University Medical Centre Rotterdam,
The Netherlands

D. Papamichael, R.A. Audisio (eds.), *Management of Colorectal Cancers in Older People*,
DOI 10.1007/978-0-85729-984-0_6, © Springer-Verlag London 2013

Introduction

The incidence of colorectal cancer increases with age and peaks around 70 years. Approximately 1 out of 20 persons older than 70 years will develop colorectal cancer [1]. Surgical resection is still the cornerstone of curative treatment of this disease. Multimodality treatment has been investigated in several randomized trials and has found its way to the national guidelines. Subsequently, on a population-based level, outcomes from both rectal and colon cancer have gradually improved. However, elderly patients did not benefit as well from the introduction of modern surgical techniques and neo- or adjuvant treatments, so that the survival gap between younger and older colorectal cancer patients is widened [2–4].

Elderly patients are underrepresented in randomized controlled trials and, when included, a selection bias is suspected as only fit individuals with a good performance are considered [5, 6]. Therefore, when developing a treatment plan for older colorectal cancer patients who have to undergo major abdominal surgery, the surgeon has to rely on guidelines, which are not evidence-based specifically for this older patient group. In fact, wide and general acceptance of evidence-based guidelines has not resulted in an improved outcome for these patients. Therefore, those guidelines, based on studies recruiting younger colorectal cancer patients, cannot automatically be applied to older patients. Importantly, the great heterogeneity in the elderly population stretches the possibilities to construct randomized controlled trials. Current clinical trial designs might be not equally applicable in the presence of the multiple comorbidities which often affect senior patients. Guidelines in geriatric oncology should also incorporate data from large, population-based cohort studies and alternative trial designs [7]. There is a difference between rectal cancer surgery and colon cancer surgery. The magnitude of the latter is much less than the first. Therefore, treatment schedules have developed differently and will be discussed separately.

Rectal Cancer

Surgery for rectal cancer should be considered major visceral surgery. The risk of developing complications rises especially after neoadjuvant treatment [8]. General complications like pulmonary and cardiovascular complications increase with age. Surgery-related complications are relatively comparable to those in younger patients [9]. However, if they do occur, the consequences are far more severe and will more often lead to postoperative mortality. The Association of Coloproctology of Great Britain and Ireland (ACPGBI) developed a nomogram based on a large population-based study [10, 11].

In a study looking at the data of the Dutch TME study, it was demonstrated that after rectal surgery, elderly had an increased postoperative mortality risk depending on age, but this risk also persisted for at least 6 months. Therefore, when reporting on postoperative mortality in elderly, mortality rates up to 6 months should be reported [9]. As shown in Fig. 6.1, analysis of population-based data at the Comprehensive Cancer Center South confirmed this finding.

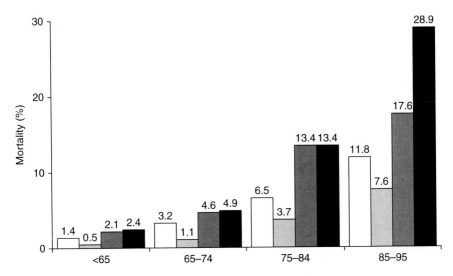

Fig. 6.1 Postoperative mortality 75 and older patients in the TME study and Comprehensive Cancer Center South study at 30 days (*white and light gray*) and 6 months (*dark gray and black*), respectively (Reprinted from Rutten et al. [9]. Copyright 2008. With permission from Elsevier)

It is clear that elderly patients receive less treatment [12]. The initial diagnostic procedures are mostly similar to the ones that usually offered to younger patients. However, elderly patients tend to receive less radiotherapy and neoadjuvant chemotherapy.

Do we have arguments that elderly have a worse oncological outcome after multi-modality treatment? In an update of the TME data, it is shown that cancer-specific mortality of elderly in the control arm which did not receive neoadjuvant radiotherapy have a worse outcome than those who have had neoadjuvant treatment; as a consequence, there are indications that elderly respond to neoadjuvant treatment and, from the TME data, it is even conceivable that elderly respond better than their younger counterparts [13, 14]. However, the overall survival remains the same. There seems to be a strong competitive risk for dying of other causes in those who received five times 5 Gy preoperatively compared to those who underwent surgery alone. We do have arguments that improved treatment involving better sequence and combination of different treatment modalities may lead to a considerable increase in survival of rectal cancer on a population-based level [15, 16]. As mentioned before, elderly patients did not seem to achieve such a significant survival improvement as younger patients did. Excess mortality overrides any beneficial effect of combined treatment modalities; it appears that elderly patients with rectal cancer are not only threatened by a local recurrence and the development of distant metastatic disease but also by the excessive mortality due to the treatment itself. Therefore, alternative therapeutic options may be worth considering for these patients. The aim to avoid major morbidity resulting from the *cancer* treatment in patients at high risk to *non-cancer*-related death should be kept in mind during multidisciplinary treatment planning. To date, however, there is no agreement on a perfect assessment tool that might assist clinicians in the selection process.

One of the most attractive alternatives is to avoid major abdominal surgery, thus avoiding complications and subsequent mortality. An interesting option to proceed is to replace intra-abdominal surgery by a local procedure. Transanal endoscopic microsurgery (TEM) may be an attractive alternative [17]. Unfortunately, there is only a small minority of elderly rectal cancer patients presenting with an early T1-rectal cancer, which could be safely treated by local excision or TEM. Recently, studies from Habr-Gama have refreshed such an interest [18, 19]. She showed that after neoadjuvant radio-chemotherapy, 25 % rectal cancer patients achieve a complete clinical remission, which seemed to be very long lasting in the majority of patients. Salvage surgery had to be performed only on a small part of these patients. The proportion of persistent complete remissions may be increased, and particularly older patients could benefit from a modified approach, perhaps in combination with advanced chemotherapy or in combination with a higher boost of radiotherapy.

The next step could be to downstage the tumor before performing a local excision. This downstaging can be achieved with radio-chemotherapy. However, it can also be achieved with five administrations of 5 Gy followed by a long waiting period before the TEM procedure is performed [20]. A different local approach proposed by a Canadian group, presently undergoing scrutiny in an ongoing Dutch study, combines endoluminal high-dose brachytherapy with external beam irradiation [21, 22].

There is no doubt that these local procedures may lead to higher local recurrence rates; however, a higher risk of local recurrence should be balanced against the increased mortality rates after major pelvic procedures in the elderly age group. If a 20 % local recurrence rate is unacceptable in younger patients, these figures may become acceptable in older rectal cancer patients due to their excessive postoperative mortality. Another interesting point is that, if a local recurrence occurs after a TEM procedure, the rectum is still enveloped within the mesorectal fascia: from the theoretical point of view, a salvage procedure should be comparable to a primary rectal cancer procedure as the surgical dissection plains are still intact. This means that further dissection along extra anatomical plains, which often leads to more blood loss and complications, might not be necessary.

Colon Cancer

The vast majority of patients presenting with colon cancer and no distant metastatic disease will undergo surgical resection. The resection rate for all age groups in stage I to III colon cancer ranges from 98 to 100 %: Even octogenarians are most frequently considered for a colonic resection [3, 17]. Different from rectal cancer, the use of neoadjuvant radiotherapy with/without chemotherapy is of limited use in colon cancer patients. Dose-limiting structures in the abdomen, like the small bowel and kidneys, prevent the administration of sufficient radiation dose that may lead to a downstaging of the primary tumor. Moreover, the predominant symptoms of colon cancer in elderly patients are chronic blood loss and anemia, and/or obstruction, with a significant risk of a complete obstruction. These life-threatening symptoms

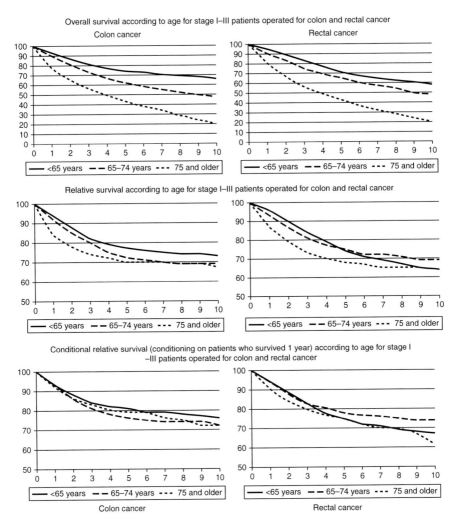

Fig. 6.2 Overall, relative, and conditional (excluding first-year mortality) survival of older and younger colon and rectal cancer patients (Reprinted from Dekker et al. [23]. With kind permission from Springer Science + Business Media)

are best treated with a surgical resection. Despite the fact that the magnitude of the surgical procedure in the case of colon cancer is much less extensive than in rectal cancer, postoperative complications may occur, leading to increased mortality rates for the elderly subgroup.

An analysis of colon and rectal cancer patients treated between 1991 and 2005 within the cancer registry of the Comprehensive Cancer Centre West (CCCW) looked at the population-based survival data for the different age groups of patients younger than 65 years, 65–74 years, and 75 years and older (Fig. 6.2). By calculating the relative survival and the conditional relative survival of patients surviving at least 1 year from surgery, the excess mortality was calculated for elderly patients. One of the key findings was that conditional relative survival, when adjusted for first-year postoperative mortality, was equal for all age groups. The remarkable conclusion was that there was no difference in colon cancer survival for each age group. The excess mortality of elderly colon cancer patients may be attributed solely to an increased mortality during the first 12 months after surgery [23]. Acute surgery, comorbidity, and postoperative complications were the most important prognosticators resulting in a 12-month mortality of almost 50 % [24]. It is reasonable to conclude that acute surgery should be avoided in elderly at all costs and swift diagnostic routes should be set in place in order to prevent obstructing conditions to become acute. It is mandatory to correct all deranged parameters and bring older patients to optimal condition before surgery is undertaken. Nutritional deficits should be corrected as well as fluid balance; medication should be optimized in agreement with the anesthetists and, when needed, the geriatric team. If acute surgery is anyway needed, the procedure should be the least traumatic as possible. Anastomosis do not leak more often in elderly patients, but they do leak more often after acute surgery, and the consequences in older colon cancer patients are more severe leading to a significantly increased postoperative mortality. Therefore, in the acute setting, a two-stage procedure aiming restoring the bowel continuity is the first and primary target; the bowel resection for therapeutic purposes can be safely postponed at a later stage [25, 26]. Surgery for colon cancer successfully leads to a long disease-free survival in elderly as in younger age groups provided that preventive measures are set in place to avoid complications and decline of the health status during the first postoperative year.

Individual Age Reflects Accumulated and Progressive Changes in the Complex System of Physiologic Response to Trauma

With the age progression, physiological changes are accumulated, and we become more vulnerable in our response to trauma. These changes will be progressive for the rest of life and will remain a threat to our capacity to respond to trauma. Major abdominal surgery will challenge different physiological response mechanisms when compared, for example, to pulmonary infection. However, like pulmonary surgery, a major abdominal surgical trauma can be life threatening to the aged patient, especially when complications occur. Age may be an indicator of limited physiological response or vulnerability to any external insult. However, the response is complex and involves numerous physiological responses depending on the type of insult. Each individual can be regarded as unique, exhibiting individual and specific changes. Unlike younger patients with more or less intact response mechanisms, older patients are uniquely depending on the combination and limitations in such physiologic responses. Therefore, individual patients cannot be compared on the basis of age alone. The difference in underlying variables is a nightmare to statisticians. However, if the sample size is large enough, a cut-off point can be identified in such a way that age becomes an independent prognostic factor for overall survival in colon and rectal cancer patients. It all depends on how detailed or selected the patient group is. As mentioned before, this is not very important for the individual patient who is dependent on his physiologic status at a given age, which also may have been influenced by factors from the past. Smoking habits, obesity, social status, education, family history, genetic, acquired factors, and many other factors determine the pace of physiological changes.

Consequences of Older Age for Surviving Colorectal Surgery

Postoperative mortality or 30-day mortality increase with age and may become a very significant factor in the elderly. In the aforementioned study, Dekker showed that excess mortality after prior colorectal surgery is significantly present until at least 12 months after surgery [16]; as previously demonstrated, the 30-day mortality is not sufficiently reflective of the true postoperative mortality in elderly. An increased risk of dying as result of the surgery persists for at least a full year. Depending on age, comorbidity, and acute need for surgery, this continuing risk may lead to a 1-year mortality of up to 70 % [8]. Apart from the physiological changes, comorbidity is also an independent adverse prognostic factor [27]. Again, it has been clearly demonstrated that chronic obstructive pulmonary disease (COPD), cardiovascular conditions, combinations of hypertension, diabetes, or renal dysfunction are responsible for an excess mortality of several 10 % [27–29] .

In a recent study from the Comprehensive Cancer Center South in the Netherlands, it was clearly confirmed that comorbidity and age are related to postoperative mortality in both colon and rectal cancer (Yvette RBM van Gestel et al., 2012, Influence of co-morbidity and age on early postoperative mortality rates in gastrointestinal cancer patients, [35]).

Relative survival figures show how improved survival has been relatively modest over the last decade in younger colon cancer patients [13]. The principles of colon cancer surgery have shown no drastic changes over the last decades whereas anesthesiology techniques have. The latter may be held responsible for at least some of the improvements noticed. Still, the use of adjuvant chemotherapy in the younger patients may have led to some change in the outcome. In elderly patients, even this modest improvement is lacking [13].

Since the introduction of TME surgery and preoperative radiotherapy, younger patients show an impressing improvement in outcome in all stages [30]. In contrast, older patients have hardly benefited from this improvement in the treatment of rectal cancer. The paper of Dekker et al. showed how the cancer-specific survival of younger and elderly patient does not differ for both colon and rectal cancer, after adjustment for age and if relative survival is also adjusted for the first 12 months after surgery. This observation leads to the conclusion that elderly patients do not have a worse cancer survival than younger patients. However, it is surprising as younger patients receive more state of the art treatment, for example, more adjuvant

Fig. 6.3 Influence of age and comorbidity on postoperative mortality (Yvette RBM van Gestel et al., 2012, unpublished data)

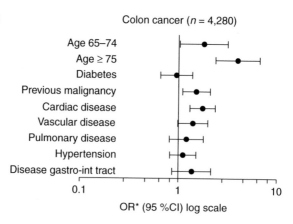

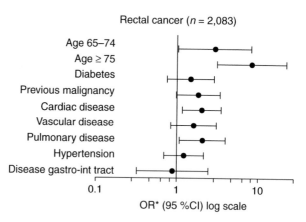

chemotherapy in colon cancer and more preoperative radiotherapy or radio-chemo therapy for rectal cancer. If they analyze the figures by stage, we notice that stage 3 elderly patients have a significantly worse prognosis than younger stage 3 colon and rectal cancer patients. This may be indicative of the fact that in these groups some of the adjuvant and neoadjuvant treatments were omitted. In rectal cancer patients, the difference is a little bit more difficult to explain as adjuvant chemotherapy is not standard in elderly or younger patients.

The other important finding was that the difference in survival could be explained by the excess mortality of elderly in the first postoperative year.

Comorbidity

There are indications that several comorbid conditions may contribute to postoperative mortality (Fig. 6.3). However, cardiopulmonary and renal dysfunctions are the strongest prognosticator for postoperative 30-day mortality. Many studies have confirmed that comorbidity has been identified as an important prognosticator. Comorbidity is not only responsible for early postoperative death but also for decreased survival in the first 6 months or even longer. The presence of comorbidity in the setting of acute surgery represents a seriously negative and possibly life-threatening combination. The acuteness of the presentation of the disease already has challenged the physiological reserve capacities; additional trauma is very likely to exhaust them further and may result into severe complications. Therefore, the principle of treating acute elderly patients should be based on minimizing any additional surgery, and more stage procedures may be preferable above a single procedure.

The dilemma when dealing with elderly colorectal cancer patients is that they do respond very well to standard cancer treatment with regard to oncological outcome, but they cope much worse with the treatment itself introducing a significant competitive risk of dying as a result of the treatment. At a population level, the magnitude of this competitive risk annihilates any of the advances made in colorectal cancer treatment. On one side, there is the discussion that too many elderly do not receive appropriate adjuvant or neoadjuvant treatment. However, introducing an even more aggressive and more toxic regiments would probably further deepen the adverse outcome for some. It would be far more cost-effective to identify those patients at risk for complicated cause. Many scoring systems ranging from physiological investigations to more psychiatric assessments have been investigated systematically [31, 32]. They have shown ability to identify the compromised less fit patient. Even so, the truly frail patient does not seem to represent a major problem, rather the majority of the seemingly healthy patients. The optimization of these patients may help to decrease the 12-month postoperative mortality. In most countries, rectal cancer patients are being discussed in a multidisciplinary oncological team. It is important to discuss these patients before commencement of any treatment strategy as the sequence of the elements of the multidisciplinary approach is critical. Similarly, all elderly colorectal cancer patients should be discussed also in a multidisciplinary team. These patients should not only have the same diagnostic procedures as the younger counterparts; they should also be assessed by a team regarding their physiological health status and with the aim of improving the health status before and during cancer treatment. For some of these patients, alternative approaches, that is, avoiding major surgical procedures could be advisable and should be openly discussed. It should also be kept in mind that none of the guidelines used in colorectal cancer patients have been validated specifically for the elderly due to their underrepresentation in such investigations. There is a gliding scale from the fit elderly patient to the geriatric patient with complex comorbidity requiring very specialistic and individualized care. On one end of the scale, the best possible oncological treatment is justified and should not be withheld. On the other side, alternative treatments, even if not indicated by any guideline, may be a more appropriate option, including no treatment.

Even after meticulous evaluation of all available options to optimize the patient for surgery to reduce its risks, counseling the older patient remains very extremely challenging. Where any improvement in oncological outcome is justified by many life years gained in the younger patients group, this is not necessarily the case for the elderly where small changes in the functional capacities may lead to drastic derangements in daily life. In general, older patients are less interested in long-term oncological outcome but more in the consequences and the impact on their daily life activities. Will they become dependent? Will they require admission to specialized residential nursing homes? This kind of information is not easily and routinely provided by surgeons; hence, the absolute need of a multidisciplinary approach which should include the patient's general physician who is better aware of the patient dependency. A careful and holistic approach is most likely to optimize organ function, and the involvement of a geriatric specialist may successfully combine all these medical, social, and psychological information about each individual patient.

Conclusions

1. Age is an independent prognostic factor; however, anagraphic age is not relevant. Instead, all physiologic changes that may have occurred are to be investigated and should be taken into account before finalizing the surgical therapeutic strategy.
2. Comorbidities are crucially important prognostic variables which should be carefully appraised and optimized before any treatment is set in place.
3. Emergency surgery is an independent major prognostic variable and should be avoided at all costs or minimized when this is not possible.
4. Elderly colorectal cancer patients represent a very heterogeneous group ranging from the very fit who are entitled to full oncological treatment, to the very frail who cannot sustain any treatment at all. Elderly patients require an individualized treatment which can only be decided after a meticulous assessment of the functional capacities.
5. Existing guidelines may be evidence based but should be critically considered they were not validated on elderly patients, most importantly on frail older patients.
6. Counseling older colorectal cancer patients should focus on the patient's perspective; this may often differ from the ordinary expectations of a younger patient.

Being the provider of the most important therapeutic option to colorectal patients, the surgeon must be fully aware that the surgical procedure in itself may lead to extremely high 12-month mortality rates. Centralization of complex cancer types has led to substantial improvement in outcomes, not only with regard to oncological results but also by reducing complications and minimizing postoperative mortality [33, 34]. The persisting risk of dying in the first 12 months after surgery for some elderly patients is considerably higher than the risk of dying from cancer. Maybe some of the more frail patients should be only treated in specialized centers where extra care is available before, during, and after surgery.

References

1. Ferlay J, Parkin DM, Steliarova-Foucher E. Estimates of cancer incidence and mortality in Europe in 2008. Eur J Cancer. 2010;46(4):765–81.
2. Quaglia A, Tavilla A, Shack L, Brenner H, Janssen-Heijnen M, Allemani C, et al. The cancer survival gap between elderly and middle-aged patients in Europe is widening. Eur J Cancer. 2009;45(6):1006–16.
3. Lemmens V, Steenbergen LV, Janssen-Heijnen M, Martijn H, Rutten H, Coebergh JW. Trends in colorectal cancer in the south of the Netherlands 1975–2007: rectal cancer survival levels with colon cancer survival. Acta Oncol. 2010;49(6):784–96.
4. Rutten H, Dulk M, Lemmens V, Nieuwenhuijzen G, Krijnen P, Jansen-Landheer M, et al. Survival of elderly rectal cancer patients not improved: analysis of population based data on the impact of TME surgery. Eur J Cancer. 2007;43(15):2295–300.
5. Townsley CA, Selby R, Siu LL. Systematic review of barriers to the recruitment of older patients with cancer onto clinical trials. J Clin Oncol. 2005;23(13):3112–24.
6. Zulman DM, Sussman JB, Chen X, Cigolle CT, Blaum CS, Hayward RA. Examining the evidence: a systematic review of the inclusion and analysis of older adults in randomized controlled trials. J Gen Intern Med. 2011;26(7):783–90.
7. Seymour MT, Thompson LC, Wasan HS, Middleton G, Brewster AE, Shepherd SF, et al. Chemotherapy options in elderly and frail patients with metastatic colorectal cancer (MRC FOCUS2): an open-label, randomised factorial trial. Lancet. 2011;377(9779):1749–59.
8. Fleming FJ, Pahlman L, Monson JR. Neoadjuvant therapy in rectal cancer. Dis Colon Rectum. 2011;54(7):901–12.
9. Rutten HJ, den Dulk M, Lemmens VE, van de Velde CJ, Marijnen CA. Controversies of total mesorectal excision for rectal cancer in elderly patients. Lancet Oncol. 2008;9(5):494–501.
10. Tan E, Tilney H, Thompson M, Smith J, Tekkis PP. The United Kingdom National Bowel Cancer Project – epidemiology and surgical risk in the elderly. Eur J Cancer. 2007;43(15):2285–94.
11. Heriot AG, Tekkis PP, Smith JJ, Cohen CR, Montgomery A, Audisio RA, et al. Prediction of postoperative mortality in elderly patients with colorectal cancer. Dis Colon Rectum. 2006;49(6):816–24.
12. van den Broek CB, Dekker JW, Bastiaannet E, Krijnen P, de Craen AJ, Tollenaar RA, et al. The survival gap between middle-aged and elderly colon cancer patients. Time trends in treatment and survival. Eur J Surg Oncol. 2011;37(10):904–12.
13. Lemmens V, van Steenbergen L, Janssen-Heijnen M, Martijn H, Rutten H, Coebergh JW. Trends in colorectal cancer in the south of the Netherlands 1975–2007: rectal cancer survival levels with colon cancer survival. Acta Oncol. 2010;49(6):784–96.
14. Rutten H, den Dulk M, Lemmens V, Nieuwenhuijzen G, Krijnen P, Jansen-Landheer M, et al. Survival of elderly rectal cancer patients not improved: analysis of population based data on the impact of TME surgery. Eur J Cancer. 2007;43(15):2295–300.
15. Birgisson H, Talback M, Gunnarsson U, Pahlman L, Glimelius B. Improved survival in cancer of the colon and rectum in Sweden. Eur J Surg Oncol. 2005;31(8):845–53.
16. Elferink MAG, van Steenbergen LN, Krijnen P, Lemmens VEPP, Rutten HJ, Marijnen CAM, et al. Marked improvements in survival of patients with rectal cancer in the Netherlands following changes in therapy, 1989–2006. Eur J Cancer. 2010;46(8):1421–9.
17. de Graaf EJ, Doornebosch PG, Tollenaar RA, Meershoek-Klein KE, de Boer AC, Bekkering FC, et al. Transanal endoscopic microsurgery versus total mesorectal excision of T1 rectal adenocarcinomas with curative intention. Eur J Surg Oncol. 2009;35(12):1280–5.
18. Habr-Gama A, Perez RO, Proscurshim I, Campos FG, Nadalin W, Kiss D, et al. Patterns of failure and survival for nonoperative treatment of stage c0 distal rectal cancer following neoadjuvant chemoradiation therapy. J Gastrointest Surg. 2006;10(10):1319–28.

19. Habr-Gama A, Perez RO, Nadalin W, Sabbaga J, Ribeiro Jr U, Silva E, Sousa Jr AH, et al. Operative versus nonoperative treatment for stage 0 distal rectal cancer following chemoradiation therapy: long-term results. Ann Surg. 2004;240(4):711–7.
20. Bokkerink GM, de Graaf EJ, Punt CJ, Nagtegaal ID, Rutten H, Nuyttens JJ, et al. The CARTS study: chemoradiation therapy for rectal cancer in the distal rectum followed by organ-sparing transanal endoscopic microsurgery. BMC Surg. 2011;11(1):34.
21. Vuong T, Belliveau PJ, Michel RP, Moftah BA, Parent J, Trudel JL, et al. Conformal preoperative endorectal brachytherapy treatment for locally advanced rectal cancer: early results of a phase I/II study. Dis Colon Rectum. 2002;45(11):1486–93.
22. Vuong T, Devic S, Podgorsak E. High dose rate endorectal brachytherapy as a neoadjuvant treatment for patients with resectable rectal cancer. Clin Oncol (R Coll Radiol). 2007;19(9):701–5.
23. Dekker JW, van den Broek CB, Bastiaannet E, van de Geest LG, Tollenaar RA, Liefers GJ. Importance of the first postoperative year in the prognosis of elderly colorectal cancer patients. Ann Surg Oncol. 2011;18(6):1533–9.
24. Gooiker GA, Dekker JW, Bastiaanet E, van der Geest LG, Merkus JW, van de Velde CJ, Tollenaar RA, Liefers GJ. Risk factors for excess mortality in the first year after curative surgery for colorectal cancer. Ann Surg Oncol. Aug;19(8):2428–34. Epub 2012 Mar 7. PubMed PMID: 22396000; PubMed Central PMCID: PMC3404283.
25. Jiang JK, Lan YT, Lin TC, Chen WS, Yang SH, Wang HS, et al. Primary vs. delayed resection for obstructive left-sided colorectal cancer: impact of surgery on patient outcome. Dis Colon Rectum. 2008;51(3):306–11.
26. Ansaloni L, Andersson RE, Bazzoli F, Catena F, Cennamo V, Di SS, et al. Guidelenines in the management of obstructing cancer of the left colon: consensus conference of the world society of emergency surgery (WSES) and peritoneum and surgery (PnS) society. World J Emerg Surg. 2010;5:29.
27. Lemmens VE, Janssen-Heijnen ML, Verheij CD, Houterman S, Repelaer van Driel OJ, Coebergh JW. Co-morbidity leads to altered treatment and worse survival of elderly patients with colorectal cancer. Br J Surg. 2005;92(5):615–23.
28. Lemmens VE, Janssen-Heijnen ML, Houterman S, Verheij KD, Martijn H, Poll-Franse L, et al. Which comorbid conditions predict complications after surgery for colorectal cancer? World J Surg. 2007;31(1):192–9.
29. Shahir MA, Lemmens VE, van de Poll-Franse LV, Voogd AC, Martijn H, Janssen-Heijnen ML. Elderly patients with rectal cancer have a higher risk of treatment-related complications and a poorer prognosis than younger patients: a population-based study. Eur J Cancer. 2006;42(17):3015–21.
30. van Gijn W, Marijnen CA, Nagtegaal ID, Kranenbarg EM, Putter H, Wiggers T, et al. Preoperative radiotherapy combined with total mesorectal excision for resectable rectal cancer: 12-year follow-up of the multicentre, randomised controlled TME trial. Lancet Oncol. 2011;12(6):575–82.
31. Kristjansson SR, Nesbakken A, Jordhoy MS, Skovlund E, Audisio RA, Johannessen HO, et al. Comprehensive geriatric assessment can predict complications in elderly patients after elective surgery for colorectal cancer: a prospective observational cohort study. Crit Rev Oncol Hematol. 2010;76(3):208–17.
32. Papamichael D, Audisio R, Horiot JC, Glimelius B, Sastre J, Mitry E, et al. Treatment of the elderly colorectal cancer patient: SIOG expert recommendations. Ann Oncol. 2009;20(1):5–16.
33. Lemmens VE, Bosscha K, van der Schelling G, Brenninkmeijer S, Coebergh JW, de Hingh IH. Improving outcome for patients with pancreatic cancer through centralization. Br J Surg. 2011;98(10):1455–62.
34. van de Poll-Franse LV, Lemmens VE, Roukema JA, Coebergh JW, Nieuwenhuijzen GA. Impact of concentration of oesophageal and gastric cardia cancer surgery on long-term population-based survival. Br J Surg. 2011;98(7):956–63.
35. van Gastel YR, Lemmens VE, de Hingh IH, Steevens J, Rutten HJ, Nieuwenhuijzen GA, van Dam RM, Siersema PD. Influance of Comorbidity and Age on 1, 2 and 3 Month Postoperative Mortality Rates in gastrointestinal Cancer Patients. Ann Surg Oncol. 2012 Sep 18. [Epub ahead of print] PubMed PMID: 22987098.

Chapter 7
Palliative Surgical Approaches for Older Patients with Colorectal Cancer

Andrew P. Zbar and Riccardo A. Audisio

Abstract Colorectal cancer is a condition of increasing age, where up to 40 % of cases present as colorectal emergencies, most notably obstruction and perforation. The adoption of screening programs in this cohort has been shown to slightly reduce these emergency presentations in high-risk cases, although screening in the elderly will have different aims than that of the rest of the population. In older patients, screening will be designed to detect cancers at an earlier stage, where polyp detection will in some cases be less important given the relationship between polyp transformation and the expected lifespan of the patient. In older patients, more palliative resections are performed with less use of adjuvant and neoadjuvant therapies, although there is no current evidence which suggests that the elderly are unsuitable for adjuvant chemotherapies or radiation protocols. A more standardized assessment of attendant comorbidities and an objective expression of a frailty index will assist in defining those patients at perioperative risk and better delineate cases at higher risk of postoperative institutionalization or who require more intensive monitoring and planned intensive care stays. The issue of colonic stenting, either as definitive therapy or as a bridge to surgery, is discussed as it applies to the elderly, suggesting that there is no overall disadvantage with stent use in cancer-specific survival and that there might be substantial cost benefit with a reduced need for stomas, a higher primary anastomosis rate and reduced length of hospital and ICU stay. The adoption of minimally invasive surgery for both colonic and rectal cancer is lagging in the elderly, where initial data suggests that perioperative mortality and morbidity is unaffected by age. Equally, the expansion of hepatic resection in

A.P. Zbar, M.D. (Lond), MBBS, FRCS (ED), FRCS (Gen), FRACS, FCCS, FSICCR (Hon)(✉)
Surgery and Transplantation, Chaim Sheba Medical Center,
Tel Hashomer, Ramat Gan, Tel Aviv 52621, Israel
e-mail: apzbar1355@yahoo.com

R.A. Audisio, M.D., FRCS
Department of Surgery, St. Helens and Knowsley Teaching Hospitals,
St Helens, Merseyside WA9 3DA, UK

D. Papamichael, R.A. Audisio (eds.), *Management of Colorectal Cancers in Older People*,   65
DOI 10.1007/978-0-85729-984-0_7, © Springer-Verlag London 2013

metastatic cases to the elderly shows that detailed patient selection is associated with good outcomes in those over 70 years of age. The question of management of the stage IV case with a minimally symptomatic (or asymptomatic) colorectal primary remains controversial, where data shows that the likelihood of the primary presenting as an emergent surgical problem is low. The use of chemo-immunotherapy and radiation in this group of elderly cases currently is under-represented and needs better definition.

Keywords Symptom management • Palliative surgery • Cancer surgery • Colorectal cancer • Older patients

Introduction

Nearly two-thirds of solid malignancies are now diagnosed in patients over 65 years of age, where the annual age-adjusted incidence of cancer shows a steady increase by some 15 % overall during the last 30 years to 450 cases per 100,000 of the population [1]. These changes are also reflected in the coincident increase in cancer-related and cancer-specific mortality in contrast with an annual decline in heart-related death rates elderly patients by about 30 % over the same time period [2, 3]. Population statistics provide a somewhat complex reasoning in the interpretation of such data where there is an increase in life expectancy as well as a true increase in cancer incidence with advancing age. In this respect, the lifetime probability of development of an invasive cancer is nearly 1 in 2 in males and 1 in 3 in females where the vast majority of the risk occurs in patients who are over 60 years of age [4].

The issues in colorectal cancer management in the elderly are complex. There needs to be international agreement concerning the estimation by surgical oncologists and multidisciplinary management teams regarding operative risk and age-related comorbidity, a comparative determination of survival limitation resultant from cancer progression in individual cases and objective considerations regarding the ancillary delivery of optimal cancer care through adjuvant and neoadjuvant therapies in this patient group. The delineation of a registerable impact of age-related comorbidity has been shown to be almost universal in this patient cohort including the end-organ impact of hypertension, diabetes, atherosclerotic disease, chronic respiratory disease, and arthritis as well as a subgroup with significant cognitive dysfunction [5–7].

Any objective assessment in the elderly should be considered against the frequent background of suboptimal surgical and adjuvant treatments in solid cancer management [8–10] and by some specialist clinicians not to incorporate older patients either into clinical trials using novel chemotherapeutic and immunotherapeutic regimens or into existing screening programs [11–13]. For whatever reason, barriers to inclusion of elderly patients in such trials has provided a paucity of data concerning their exact role in standard clinical presentations and include variations in physician perception regarding the safety of surgical therapies, protocol eligibility criteria (where many protocols create age-related exclusion criteria for recruitment), comorbidity exclusions, assumptions regarding the potential tolerability of treatments, and the perceived lack of social support networks necessary for optimal follow-up or for the ability to withstand treatment-related side effects requiring such support [14, 15]. In this regard, it is known in colorectal cancer that many elderly patients tolerate adjuvant chemotherapeutic regimes without a significant increase in severe chemotherapy-related toxicity, although there is a higher incidence in older patients of chemotherapy-related hospital admissions during treatment for anemia, diarrhea, and dehydration [16, 17].

This chapter assesses the inherent differences from the general population in colorectal cancer presentation in the elderly, the general approaches clinicians currently adopt toward operative management risk assessment, the use of colonic stenting in older patients either as a definitive palliation in acute obstruction or as a bridge to curative resection, and the changing paradigm of treatment in those presenting with stage IV and specifically hepatic metastatic disease from colorectal cancer.

Colorectal Cancer Presentation in the Elderly: Is It Different?

Data from the Association of Coloproctology of Great Britain and Ireland (the ACPGBI) shows an age-adjusted increase in mortality in colorectal cancer where patients between 65 and 74 years have a 1.8-fold greater likelihood of death, those between 75 and 84 years a 3.5-fold increase, and those >85 years a fivefold increase in death rates following elective colorectal resection [18]. This data is, however, unadjusted for ASA grade, cancer site, or stage at presentation where the Colorectal Cancer Collaborative Group has previously shown that older patients with colorectal cancer have as expected a higher baseline comorbidity and more advanced disease stage and undergo more frequent emergency surgeries [19]. Elderly patients present more often than their younger counterparts as colorectal emergencies (most notably, as obstruction and/or perforation), where these types of presentations occur in up to 40 % of cases. In this setting, there is a considerably higher likelihood of palliative surgeries and a lower utilization of adjuvant and neoadjuvant therapies [20]. In this regard, there are only minimal data that the institution of a definitive screening program in elderly patients actually impacts this acute presentation where Davies et al. [21] have shown in the UK that the introduction of a fast-track service which attempts to meet the 2-week target of clinical consultation introduced in July 2000 [22] has resulted in a trend toward fewer emergency presentations after target institution. This approach did not specifically target elderly cases and showed only a modest reduction in emergency presentation by the routine use of a flexible sigmoidoscopic service (4.1 % reduction) where only half of all colorectal cancers were diagnosed within the instituted fast-track system.

The potential advantages of such an approach should reduce the likelihood of emergency surgery in patients over the age of 80 years if there is a definitive change in screening criteria based on increasing the age limit [23, 24]. In elderly cases, only

4–6 % of colorectal lesions are Dukes' stage A compared with 9.2 % of the general population in two large UK studies [25, 26], although a balance needs to be provided between the aims of colonoscopic screening in older patients where the goals of polyp detection and their progression over considerable time and the benefits of endoscopic polypectomy need to be assessed in terms of expected life expectancy from other age-related illnesses. Here, the distinction should be made in the elderly cohort between cancer prevention through polyp detection and endoscopic polypectomy treatment and early disease detection before a definitive screening program in the elderly can be nationally adopted even when the absolute risk for developing colorectal cancer is highest in this age group. This balance must also incorporate the real risks of colonoscopy-related morbidity and mortality in very old cases [27] as well as evidence showing lower procedural completion rates and higher rates of inadequate bowel preparation [28]. Even though the prevalence rates of colorectal neoplasia are high in this group, there appears to be smaller gains in life expectancy when compared with younger patient cohorts even when adjusted for life expectancy. This elective concept is separable from the aim of diminishing the likelihood of acute emergency colorectal presentations in such cases.

Comprehensive Geriatric Assessment (CGA) in Colorectal Cancer

A series of structured questionnaires have been recently established and validated for elderly patients with solid malignancies undergoing surgery incorporating the specific functional, mental, and social parameters which uniquely affect cancer-related outcome in this unique patient group [29]. In this regard, Audisio and colleagues in collaboration with the International Society of Geriatric Oncology (SIOG) and with geriatricians have developed the PACE (preoperative assessment of cancer in the elderly) questionnaire for rapid patient risk determination showing that 83 % of patients have at least one relatively important comorbid condition and that only two-thirds of cases have acceptable preoperative functional and mental status [30, 31]. Following adjustment for age, sex, and type of cancer, most of the PACE parameters have been shown to be significantly associated with other comorbidity indices where a multivariate analysis has identified that an instrumental activity of daily living index (IADL), a brief fatigue index and the American Society of Anesthesia (ASA) grade are independent risk factors predicting for poor postoperative outcomes [32–34]. It is anticipated that a more intensive geriatric assessment will better define an estimate of remaining life expectancy, functional reserve, and treatment tolerance as well as assist in outlining individual barriers to adjuvant treatment and hospital discharge.

Universal acceptance of standardized parameters are of major clinical importance in this clinical setting where preoperative disturbances of the IADL, fatigue, and performance status lead to a 50 % increase in the incidence of both postoperative complications [35] and extended hospital stay [36]. Incorporating these questionnaires prospectively into multidimensional assessments will provide comparability of cancer-specific outcome data between elderly and younger patient groups in specific cancers and will assist in the identification of variability in preoperative staging and factors which limit the use of postoperative adjuvant therapies. Although these instruments require further validation and dissection, frailty as an index has been independently shown in the Netherlands study to be a major risk factor for institutionalization, mortality, and a decline in physical functioning after major cancer surgery in population-based patient cohorts [37], although its discriminatory ability to identify patients with a heightened vulnerability to adverse health events as part of a multisystem reduction in functional reserve capacity remains controversial [38].

The Place of Colonic Stenting

The issues (and opportunities) available to all patients with colorectal cancer should also be a routine part of oncologic practice in the elderly, including access to laparoscopic and robotic technology, emergency stenting (where appropriate), and utilization of adjuvant and neoadjuvant therapies. Older patients presenting with obstructive colorectal cancer have a death rate three times higher than that of younger cohorts presenting as colonic emergencies where typically the older case undergoes a diverting stoma [39] and where at least half the patients will never undergo stoma reversal. There is no current available data where age is an independent factor concerning outcome of stented versus unstented patients and stenting studies have essentially been nonrandomized. Here, comparisons have been made with palliative surgery only where the indications for their use, (namely, the bridge approach toward curative resection versus the definitive palliative approach) have not been adequately compared [40, 41]. Table 7.1 shows recent available data concerning stent use in obstructive settings.

In the bridging situation, successful primary anastomosis rates appear higher in the stented group with an acceptably low leakage rate (3 % stent vs. 11 % with no stent) along with a shorter hospital stay and a reduced surgical intensive care unit utilization although there is little available information concerning the effect of a bridge on overall cancer-specific outcomes [43, 44]. The exact place of stenting remains controversial where the complication rate (late perforation) has been unexpectedly high in the Dutch Stent-in-1 trial necessitating early trial closure [48, 49]. Cost analyses comparing stents with surgery have shown that stenting results in 23 % fewer operative procedures per patient (1.01 vs. 1.32 operations per patient) with an 83 % reduction in stoma formation (7 % vs. 43 %) and a lower procedure-related mortality (5 % vs. 11 %) and a lower mean cost per patient where stenting options were used as the first line of treatment [50]. The most recent data from China comparing mortality, stoma avoidance, and short-term survival specifically in the elderly where stents were compared with acute surgery matched for tumor distribution and comorbidity, showed a successful stent deployment rate of 91 % with a higher rate of primary anastomosis (79 % vs. 47 %; $P=0.002$), and a comparable mortality and morbidity between groups [46]. In this presentation, there is considerable

Table 7.1 Reported data concerning colonic stent use as a bridge to resection and as definitive palliation in colonic obstruction

Author (year) [ref.]	Number	Trial design	Success (%)	Mortality (%)	LOHS	Stoma use	Compl (%)
Law et al. (2003) [40]	61	NRT/Open Bridge	96.7	13.3 vs. 25.8	Reduced	13.3 vs. 48.4	NS
Carne et al. (2004) [43, 44]	44	NRT/Open	88	0	Reduced	8 vs. 63.2	–
Ng et al. (2006) [41]	60	NRT/Open Bridge	95	5 vs. 12.5	Reduced	5 vs. 27.5	Perf (5 %)
Xinopulos et al. (2004) [42]	15	Open label	93.3	–	28 days		Migration (6.7)
Trompetas et al. (2010) [45]	12	Open label	83.3	36	NS	16.7	Perf (8)
Guo et al. (2011) [46][a]	92	NRT/Open Bridge plus definitive	91	2.9 vs. 18.9	NS	21 vs. 53	Perf (2.9 %)
Selinger et al. (2011) [47]	96	Open label	83.3	2.5	NS	–	26.3 % overall complications

Studies were performed as a bridge to resection or as definitive treatment

LOHS length of hospital stay, *NRT* nonrandomized trial (stent *vs.* open surgery or stoma), *DD* delayed dehiscence, *Compl* complications, *Perf* perforation, *NS* not stated

[a]The only available study specifically used in elderly case

work yet to be done where age is an independent factor in the decision making for acute stents particularly as the site of the obstruction does not appear to play a factor in outcome [47] and where longer-term palliation is best achieved in colonic cases rather than in tumors creating extracolonic obstruction [45]. The aims in elderly cases may be different when compared with their younger cohort, where the presence of a stoma will leave older cases with the dual burden of recovery from acute surgery and the social impact of managing a stoma. There does not appear to be a specific difference in overall survival between patients undergoing preoperative colonic decompression and those going straight to colonic surgery [51] where in many cases, overall survival is not a measure of colonic cancer advancement but rather of attendant life-threatening comorbidities [52].

The Changing Paradigm of Management of Stage IV Colorectal Cancer in the Elderly

Many collective retrospective series have shown that the short-term morbidity and cancer-specific survival are equivalent in elderly patients undergoing elective colorectal resection when compared with younger cohorts [53–61]. Recent comparative but nonrandomized data clearly shows advantage for older patients in the laparoscopic approach akin to younger cases, with significantly less blood loss when compared with open surgery and an overall faster recovery rate [62, 63] and without any specific age-related effect in elderly cases on perioperative mortality [64] or upon short- or medium-term outcomes [65]. The utilization of laparoscopic surgery in more clinically advanced colonic cancers presenting in older patients requires larger studies [66] where there might be a higher incidence of preclusive prior abdominal surgery [67] and differential adverse effects of laparoscopic conversion [68]. For rectal cancer, the principal issues include the more routine use of neoadjuvant therapy combined with a laparoscopic approach. With regard to the extended role of laparoscopic and robotic surgery in the elderly with rectal cancer, there is a paucity of data. Perioperative morbidity is affected by the inherent operative learning curve [69] as well as by the higher comorbidity observed in older patients [70]. In one of the few available studies assessing the impact of age on elective laparoscopic rectal surgery, Akiyoshi and colleagues compared 44 patients over the age of 75 years with 228 younger patients undergoing elective laparoscopic rectal resection as well as with 43 elderly patients having open rectal resections [71], showing no differences between the laparoscopic groups in terms of operating times, estimated blood loss, or postoperative complication rate, but with a marked reduction in blood loss when compared with the open group despite a substantial increase in operating time when the laparoscopic approach was adopted. Although in this study the incidence of postoperative complications was less in the elderly laparoscopic group when compared with the open elderly group, these differences did not reach statistical significance. The implication is that laparoscopy should not be denied to appropriate patients because of their chronological age. It is anticipated that tumor size, operator experience, and tumor location as well as intrinsic "pelvic" factors such as gender and body habitus and mass index are more important than age-related nonsurgical factors in determining the success rate of laparoscopic rectal resection [72]. Further factors involved in patient outcome which are more age-dependent show a greater incidence of postoperative renal failure and in-hospital deaths where surgery is emergent in elderly patients and where social considerations such as admission to hospital from a nursing facility correlated with higher rates of in-hospital mortality [73]. In these patients, it is accepted that the length of the procedure in these circumstances, the presence of significant postoperative complications, and the need for perioperative blood transfusion predict for the 6-month postoperative mortality [74].

Table 7.2 shows the outcome specifically in elderly cases of hepatectomy for colorectal metastases. The overall indications for hepatic resection in colorectal cancer metastases are increasing and are currently in a state of flux. The advancements in operative technique extend to the elderly where there are acceptable postoperative complication rates from formal hepatectomy [75, 77–84] and where there is an increasing older cohort who can be considered suitable for hepatic resection. Some of these studies are relatively difficult to interpret because they do not adequately list the range of comorbid illnesses [80] or stratify cases and because there are different extents of hepatic metastatic disease in the different age groupings. This may also partly explain the variable rates of use of neoadjuvant chemotherapy in the various age ranges. Currently, in the age of modern chemotherapy, the contraindications to formal hepatectomy in older patients are similar to younger cases, including >3 metastases, the presence of bilobar disease, concomitant extrahepatic disease, and failure to use postoperative chemotherapeutic regimens.

In colorectal cancer patients presenting with advanced (stage IV) disease, there are a range of potential options for a challenging set of problems. For rectal cancer specifically, these include extirpative resection, diversion, stenting and laser, or argon beam photocoagulation with the goals of management including symptom improvement, enhancement of quality of life, and provision of patient comfort [85]. In those patients deemed incurable by virtue of metastatic disease or local invasion which precludes margin-negative resection emphasis is on symptom-based quality-of-life parameters. In those patients primarily presenting with sciatic nerve pain, bilateral hydronephrosis, extensive sacral involvement, bilateral leg edema, and associated widespread intraperitoneal disease, the likelihood of negative circumferential margins is remote with considerable extirpative morbidity [86–88]. The commonest clinical presentations requiring palliative treatment in such cases are obstruction and bleeding and in the case of rectal cancer, pain and discharge [89], where surgical intervention does not appear to confer survival advantage. This has been supplemented by a German study showing that at least two-thirds of palliated patients will not require any further surgery [90].

Up to one quarter of patients with stage IV colorectal cancer will present with obstructive symptoms [87], although the most common symptom in these patients is bleeding [89, 90]. As noted, comparative stenting where appropriate shows 19 % of stented patients with minimal postoperative mortality versus a 32 % complication

Table 7.2 Outcomes of hepatic resection in the elderly for metastatic disease of colorectal cancer

Author (year) [ref.]	Number	Hepatectomy type	Morbidity (%)	Mortality (%)	Survival (%)	
Cescon et al. (2003) [75]	122	>70 years	39.1	–	64.2	3-year
		<70 years	21.7	2	53.9	
Menon et al. (2006) [76]	517	>70 years 111 MR	31	7.9	59	
		<70 years 374 MR	33	5.4	57	
Mazzoni et al. (2007) [77]	197	>70 years	16.3	3	30	5-year
		<70 years	14.6	2.1	38	
Figueras et al. (2007) [78]	648	>70 years	41	8	48	3-year
		<70 years	34	3	62	
Di Liguori-Carino et al. (2008) [79]	178	57.5 % MR	38.5	4.9	43.2	3-year
Adam et al. (2010) [80]	7,764	Less MR >70 years	32.3	3.8	57.1	3-year
		<70 years	28.7	1.6	60.2	

MR major resection, *NS* not stated

rate in the operative group which has a 5 % mortality [91]. In those palliated cases, one further German study has shown that most patients do not require any further surgical treatment [92] although this must be balanced against the incidence of subsequent stent complications despite satisfactory deployment, namely, bleeding, malposition, occlusion, migration, and late perforation. Low-level deployment of a stent as a palliation is associated in some patients with extrusion, incomplete stent expansion, incontinence, and morbid tenesmus [93]. Occlusion may more often than not be treated with endoscopic redeployment of a "piggy-back" stent, and bleeding can usually be controlled by endoscopic electrocoagulation and a very long segment with angulation may necessitate a colostomy rather than the risks of stent-related perforation [94]. In selected cases, these colostomies may be performed laparoscopically with minimal attendant morbidity although this can be difficult to perform safely when the colon is massively dilated. In those cases where palliative resectional surgery is performed, there is a higher incidence of stoma-related complications [95].

For bleeding, palliative options include Nd:YAG laser ablation which may also be used for tumor regrowth following stent placement [96]. Repeated treatments are required although the success rates are high with a moderate symptom-free interval of about 6 months. Complications occur in 2–15 % of cases, most of which are minor with rare incidences of perforation [97]; however, this treatment is often not successful in long-segment or circumferential tumors or in those with marked colonic angulation. The alternative here is argon plasma coagulation for fulguration; although it offers only minimal tissue depth penetration (so that perforation is rare), it is easier to use than the laser as well as being cheaper and more portable. Those presenting with pain and bleeding are more suitable for palliative irradiation with a median duration of response of 6–9 months [98] although there is no impact on survival. In selected cases where there is also metastatic disease, transanal endoscopic microsurgery can be effective as an entirely palliative approach [99].

The final controversial area of management concerns patients who present with advanced inoperable disease with an in situ relatively asymptomatic colorectal primary. Here, the management is controversial and relies on an assessment as to whether the primary is likely to become symptomatic. Traditionally, these cases have been treated with preemptive resection to deal with potential symptoms necessitating urgent treatment although this has not shown specific survival benefit [100, 101]. In an assessment of patients undergoing primary chemotherapy in such a setting comparing some of those undergoing resection of the primary tumor and those where resection of the primary tumor was deferred, Tebutt et al. showed no real difference in the groups in the subsequent incidence of obstruction, perforation, bleeding, or fistula formation [102]. In a similar study, Scoggins and colleagues [103] showed that <10 % required emergent operative intervention where chemotherapy was the primary and only treatment modality with a similar finding noted by Poultsides et al. [101]. Data are nonrandomized, and this approach still remains controversial where some have demonstrated slight median survival advantage when the primary is resected [104, 105] and where independent prognostic factors directly affecting survival have included colectomy, secondary curative attempts at surgery, exclusive liver metastases, and the absence of a need for colonic stenting [106, 107]. This data must be assessed against substantial morbidity and mortality in these high-risk cases, particularly in patients with locally advanced rectal cancer (pT4, expected R2 resection) undergoing palliative resections as well as in those with a hepatic tumor load exceeding 50 % of the hepatic volume [108]. In this setting, where Bevacizumab is utilized, there is a recorded incidence of spontaneous colonic tumor perforation (in the order of 2 %) [109] which would be avoided by primary resection, although this anti-VEGF antibody is often not utilized in many elderly patients because of the relative risk of acute cardiovascular complications [110].

Conclusions

Elderly patients frequently have not been specified in the randomized assessment of palliative treatments for advanced colorectal cancer. They are more likely to present with colorectal emergencies where the perioperative mortality and morbidity is high and where there is a frequent use of stomas which are often not reversed. In this setting, many do not receive optimal postoperative adjuvant therapy. The management of impending obstruction has shifted in selected cases toward endoscopic stenting although there is a moderately high rate of serious complications which are not well tolerated in advanced age, particularly when there is a high attendant comorbidity. Palliation for bleeding and fistula is still resection in most cases although some locally advanced rectal tumors can be effectively treated by endoscopic laser therapy, fulguration, or palliative local excision. Controversy still exists concerning the patient who presents with advanced metastatic disease with an in situ primary tumor which itself provides very little in the way of symptoms. In these cases, most would still advocate primary excision where the response to neoadjuvant chemotherapy is a little unpredictable [111–113] and where there is a presumptive guess by the clinician of the likelihood of significant symptoms requiring semi-emergent surgery although the few studies available suggest that the likelihood of acute colorectal events necessitating urgent surgery are uncommon during the patient's life span [114].

References

1. Jernal A, Murray T, Samuels A, Ghafoor A, Ward E, Thun MJ. Cancer statistics 2003. CA Cancer J Clin. 2003;53:5–26.
2. Davis DL, Dinse GE, Hoel DG. Decreasing cardiovascular disease and increasing cancer among whites in the United States from 1973 through 1987: good news and bad news. JAMA. 1984;271:431–7.
3. Leading causes of death in the United States, 1973 vs 1999. J Natl Cancer Inst 2002;94:1742.
4. Gómez Portilla A, Martínez de Lecea C, Cendoya I, Olobarría I, Martin E, Magrach L, Romero E, Cortés J, Muriel J, Márquez A, Kvadatze M. Prevalence and treatment of oncologic disease in the elderly – an impending challenge. Rev Esp Enferm Dis. 2008;11:706–15.
5. Yancik R, Havlik RJ, Wesley MN, et al. Cancer and comorbidity in older patients: a descriptive profile. Ann Epidemiol. 1996;6:399–412.
6. Yancik R, Ganz PA, Varricchio CG, Conley B. Perspectives on comorbidity and cancer in older patients: approaches to expand the knowledge base. J Clin Oncol. 2001;19:1147–51.
7. Read WL, Tierney RM, Page NC, Costas I, Govindan R, Spitznagel ELJ, Piccirillo JF. Differential prognostic impact of comorbidity. J Clin Oncol. 2004;22:3099–103.
8. Sekue I, Fukuda X, Kumitoh H, Saijo N. Cancer chemotherapy in the elderly. Jpn J Clin Oncol. 1998;28:463–73.
9. Wasil T, Lichtman SM, Gupta V, Rush S. Radiation therapy in cancer patients 80 years of age or older. Am J Clin Oncol. 2000;23:526–30.
10. Audisio RA, Bozzetti F, Gennari R, Jaklitsch MT, Koperna T, Longo WE, Wiggers T, Zbar A. The surgical management of elderly cancer patients: recommendations of the SIOG surgical task force. Eur J Cancer. 2004;40:926–38.
11. Trimble EL, Carter CL, Cain D, Freidlin B, Ungerleider RS, Friedman MA. Representation of older patients in cancer treatment trials. Cancer. 1994;74:2208–14.
12. Townsley CA, Selby R, Siu LL. Systematic review of barriers to the recruitment of older patients with cancer onto clinical trials. J Clin Oncol. 2005;23:3112–24.
13. Aapro MS, Köhne CH, Cohen HJ, Extermann M. Never too old? Age should not be a barrier to enrolment in cancer clinical trials. Oncologist. 2005;10:198–204.
14. Ficorella C, Cannita K, Ricevuto E. The adjuvant therapy of colonic carcinoma in old age. Minerva Med. 1999;90:232–3.
15. Aparicio T, Navazesh A, Boutron I, Bouarioua N, Chosidow D, Mion M, Choudat L, Sobhani I, Mentre F, Soule JC. Half of elderly patients routinely treated for colorectal cancer receive a sub-standard treatment. Crit Rev Oncol Hematol. 2009;71:249–57.

16. Reddy N, Yu J, Fakih MG. Toxicities and survival among octogenarians and nonagenarians with colorectal cancer treated with chemotherapy or concurrent chemoradiation therapy. Clin Colorectal Cancer. 2007;6:362–6.

17. Bouvier A-M, Jooste V, Bonnetain F, Cottet V, Bizollon M-H, Bernard M-P, Faivre J. Adjuvant treatments do not alter the quality of life in elderly patients with colorectal cancer: a population-based study. Cancer. 2008;113:879–86.

18. Tekkis PP, Poloniecki JD, Thompson MR, Stamatakis JD. ACPGBI Colorectal Cancer Study 2002: Part A – unadjusted outcomes. Part B – Risk adjusted outcomes. The ACPGBI colorectal cancer model. www.ncbi.nlm.nih.gov/pmc/articles/PMC1079964

19. Colorectal Cancer Collaborative Group. Surgery for colorectal cancer in elderly patients. Lancet. 2000;356:968–74.

20. Koperna T, Kisser M, Schulz F. Emergency surgery for colon cancer in the aged. Arch Surg. 1997;132:1032–7.

21. Davies RJ, Collins CD, Vickery CJ, Eyre-Brook I, Welbourn R. Reduction in the proportion of patients with colorectal cancer presenting as an emergency following the introduction of fast-track flexible sigmoidoscopy: a three-year prospective observational study. Colorectal Dis. 2004;6:265–7.

22. NHS Executive. Referral guidelines for suspected cancer. Department of Health London 1999; HSC: 241.

23. Clark AJ, Stockton D, Elder A, Wilson RG, Dunlop MG. Assessment of outcomes after colorectal cancer resection in the elderly as a rationale for screening and early detection. Br J Surg. 2004;91:1345–51.

24. Lin OS, Kozarek RA, Schembre DB, Ayub K, Gluck M, Drennan F, Soon M-S, Rabeneck L. Screening colonoscopy in very elderly patients: prevalence of neoplasia and estimated impact on life expectancy. JAMA. 2006;295:2357–65.

25. The consultant surgeons and pathologists of the Lothian and Borders Health Branch. Lothian and borders large bowel cancer project: immediate outcome after surgery. Br J Surg. 1995;82:888–90.

26. Hardcastle JD, Chamberlain JO, Robinson MH, Moss SM, Amar SS, Balfour TW, et al. Randomized controlled trial of faecal-occult-blood screening for colorectal cancer. Lancet. 1996;348:1472–7.

27. Clarke GA, Jacobson BC, Hammett RJ, Carr-Locke DL. The indications, utilization and safety of gastrointestinal endoscopy in an extremely elderly patient cohort. Endoscopy. 2001;33:580–4.

28. Ure T, Dehghan K, Vernava III AM, Longo WE, Andrus CA, Daniel GI. Colonoscopy in the elderly: low risk, high yield. Surg Endosc. 1995;9:505–8.

29. Maas HA, Janssen-Heijnen ML, Olde-Rikkert MG, et al. Comprehensive geriatric assessment and its clinical impact in oncology. Eur J Cancer. 2007;43:2161–9.

30. Pope D, Ramesh H, Gennari R, et al. Pre-operative assessment of cancer in the elderly (PACE): a comprehensive assessment of underlying characteristics of elderly cancer patients prior to elective surgery. Surg Oncol. 2006;15:189–97.

31. PACE participants, Audisio RA, Pope D, Ramesh HS, Gennari R, van Leeuwen BL, West C, Corsini G, Maffezzini M, Hoekstra HJ, Mobarak D, Bozzetti F, Colledan M, Wildiers H, Stotter A, Capewell A, Marshall E. Shall we operate? preoperative assessment in elderly cancer patients (PACE) can help. A SIOG surgical task force prospective study. Crit Rev Oncol Hematol. 2008;65:156–63.

32. Lawton MP, Brody EM. Assessment of older people: self-maintaining and instrumental activities of daily living. Gerontologist. 1969;9:179–86.

33. Mendoza TR, Wang XS, Cleeland CS, et al. The rapid assessment of fatigue severity in cancer patients: use of the brief fatigue inventory. Cancer. 1999;85:1186–96.

34. Audisio RA, van Leeuwen B. When reporting on older patients with cancer, frailty information is needed. Ann Surg Oncol. 2011;18:4–5.

35. Kristjansson SR, Nesbakken A, Jordhoy MS, Skovlund E, Audisio RA, Johannessen HO, Bakka A, Wyller TB. Comprehensive geriatric assessment can predict complications in elderly patients after elective surgery for colorectal cancer: a prospective observational cohort study. Crit Rev Oncol Hematol. 2010;76:208–17.

36. Kristjansson SR, Farinella E, Gaskell S, Audisio RA. Surgical risk and post-operative complications in older unfit cancer patients. Cancer Treat Rev. 2009;35:499–502.

37. Schuurmans H, Steverink N, Lindenberg S, et al. Old or frail: what tells us more? J Gerontol A Biol Sci Med Sci. 2004;59:M962–5.

38. Martin FC, Brighton P. Frailty: different tools for different purposes? Age Ageing. 2008;37: 129–31.

39. Pavlidis TE, Marakis G, Ballas K, et al. Safety of bowel resection for colorectal surgical emergency in the elderly. Colorectal Dis. 2006;8:657–62.

40. Law WL, Choi HK, Chu KW. Comparison of stenting with emergency surgery as palliative treatment for obstructing primary left-sided colorectal cancer. Br J Surg. 2003;90: 1429–33.

41. Ng KC, Law WL, Lee YM, et al. Self expanding metallic stents as a bridge to surgery versus emergency resection for obstructing left sided colorectal cancer: a case-matched study. J Gastrointest Surg. 2006;10:798–803.

42. Xinopoulos D, Dimitroulopoulos D, Theodosopoulos T, Tsamakidis K, Bitsakou G, Plataniotis G, Gontikakis M, Kontis M, Paraskevas I, Vassilobpoulos P, Paraskevas F. Stenting or stoma creation for patients with inoperable malignant colonic obstructions. Surg Endosc. 2004;18:421–6.

43. Carne PW, Frye JN, Robertson GM, Frizelle FA. Stents or open operation for palliation of colorectal cancer: a retrospective, cohort study of perioperative outcome and long-term survival. Dis Colon Rectum. 2004;47:1455–61.

44. Trompetas V. Emergency management of malignant acute left-sided colonic obstruction. Ann R Coll Surg Engl 2008;90:181–6.

45. Trompetas V, Saunders M, Gossage J, Anderson H. Shortcomings in colonic stenting to palliate large bowel obstruction from extracolonic malignancies. Int J Colorectal Dis. 2010;25:851–4.

46. Guo MG, Feng Y, Zheng Q, Di JZ, Wang Y, Fan YB, Huang XY. Comparison of self-expanding metal stents and urgent surgery for left-sided malignant colonic obstruction in elderly patients. Dig Dis Sci. 2011;56(9):2706–10. doi:10.1007/s10620-011-1648-4.

47. Selinger CP, Ramesh J, Martin DF. Long-term success of colonic stent insertion is influenced by indication but not by length of stent or site of obstruction. Int J Colorectal Dis. 2011;26:215–8.

48. VanHooft JE, Fockens P, Marinelli AW, et al. Premature closure of the Dutch Stent-in I study. Lancet. 2006;368:1573–4.

49. Audisio RA, Zbar AP, Johnson FE. Clinical trials for colonic stents. Lancet. 2007; 369(9557):188–9.

50. Targownik LE, Spiegel BM, Sack J, et al. Colonic stent vs. Emergency surgery for management of acute left-sided malignant colonic obstruction: a decision analysis. Gastrointest Endosc. 2004; 60:865–74.

51. Tilney HS, Lovegrove RE, Purkayastha S, et al. Comparison of colonic stenting, open surgery for malignant large bowel obstruction. Surg Endosc. 2007;21:225–33.

52. Saida Y, Sumiyama Y, Nagao J, Uramatsu M. Long-term prognosis of preoperative bridge to surgery expandable metallic stent insertion for obstructive colorectal cancer comparison with emergency operation. Dis Colon Rectum. 2003;46:S44–9.

53. Shankar A, Taylor I. Treatment of colorectal cancer in patients aged over 75. Eur J Surg Oncol. 1998;24:391–5.

54. Catena F, Pasqualini E, Tonini V, Avanzolini A, Campione O. Emergency surgery of colorectal cancer in patients older than 80 years of age. Ann Ital Chir. 2002;73:173–80.

55. Au HJ, Mulder KE, Fields AL. Systematic review of management of colorectal cancer in elderly patients. Clin Colorectal Cancer. 2003;3:165–71.

56. Fietkau R, Zettl H, Klöcking S, Kundt G. Incidence, therapy and prognosis of colorectal cancer in different age groups. A population-based cohort study of the Rostock Cancer Registry. Strahlenther Onkol. 2004;180:478–87.

57. Chiappa A, Zbar AP, Bertani E, Biffi R, Luca F, Pace U, Viale G, Pruneri G, Orecchia R, Lazzari R, Biella F, Grassi C, Zampino G, Fazio N, Della Vigna P, Andreoni L, Andreoni B. Surgical treatment of advanced colorectal cancer in the elderly. Chir Ital. 2005;57:589–96.

58. Richter P, Milanowski W, Bucki K, Kubisz A, Nowak W. Age as a prognostic factor in colorectal cancer treatment. Przegl Lek. 2005;62:1440–3.

59. Heriot AG, Tekkis PP, Smith JJ, Cohen CR, Montgomery A, Audisio RA, Thompson MR, Stamatakis JD. Prediction of postoperative mortality in elderly patients with colorectal cancer. Dis Colon Rectum. 2006;49:816–24.

60. Isobe H, Takasu N, Mizutani M, Kimura W. Management of colorectal cancer in elderly patients over 80 years old. Nippon Ronen Igakkai Zasshi. 2007;44:599–605.

61. Basili G, Lorenzetti L, Biondi G, Preziuso E, Angrisano C, Carnesecchi P, Roberto E, Goletti O. Colorectal cancer in the elderly. Is there a role for safe and curative surgery? ANZ J Surg. 2008;78:466–70.

62. Chautard J, Alves A, Zalinski S, Bretagnol F, Valleur P, Panis Y. Laparoscopic colorectal surgery in elderly patients: a matched case-control study in 178 patients. J Am Coll Surg. 2008; 206:255–60.

63. Pinto RA, Ruiz D, Edden Y, Weiss EG, Nogueras JJ, Wexner SD. How reliable is laparoscopic colorectal surgery compared with laparotomy for octogenarians? Surg Endosc. 2011; 25:2692–8.

64. Fiscon V, Portale G, Migliorini G, Frigo F. Laparoscopic resection of colorectal cancer in elderly patients. Tumori. 2010;96:704–8.

65. Robinson CN, Balentine CJ, Marshall CL, Wilks JA, Anaya D, Artinyan A, Berger DH, Albo D. Minimally invasive surgery improves short-term outcomes in elderly colorectal cancer patients. J Surg Res. 2011;166:182–8.

66. Verheijen PM, Stevenson AR, Lumley JW, Clark AJ, Stitz RW, Clark DA. Laparoscopic resection of advanced colorectal cancer. Br J Surg. 2011;98:427–30.

67. Nozaki I, Kubo Y, Kurita A, Ohta K, Aogi K, Tanada M, Takashima S. Laparoscopic colectomy for colorectal cancer patients with previous abdominal surgery. Hepatogastroenterology. 2008;55:943–6.

68. Casillas S, Delaney CP, Senagore AJ, Brady K, Fazio VW. Does conversion of a laparoscopic colectomy adversely affect patient outcome? Dis Colon Rectum. 2004;47:1680–5.

69. Bege T, Lelong B, Esterni B, Turrini O, Guiramand J, Francon D, Mokart D, Houvenaeghel G, Giovannini M, Delpero JR. The learning curve for the laparoscopic approach to conservative mesorectal excision for rectal cancer: lessons drawn from a single institution's experience. Ann Surg. 2010;251:249–53.

70. Del Rio P, Dell'Abate P, Gomes B, Fumagalli M, Papadia C, Coruzzi A, Leonardi F, Pucci F, Sianesi M. Analysis of risk factors for complications in 262 cases of laparoscopic colectomy. Ann Ital Chir. 2010;81:21–30.

71. Akiyoshi T, Kuroyanagi H, Oya M, Konishi T, Fukuda M, Fujimoto Y, Ueno M, Yamaguchi T. Short-term outcomes of laparoscopic rectal surgery for primary rectal cancer in elderly patients: is it safe and beneficial? J Gastrointest Surg. 2009;13:1614–8.

72. Ogiso S, Yamaguchi T, Hata H, Fukuda M, Ikai I, Yamato T, Sakai Y. Evaluation of factors affecting the difficulty of laparoscopic anterior resection for rectal cancer: "narrow pelvis" is not a contraindication. Surg Endosc. 2011;25:1907–12.

73. Kurian A, Suryadevara S, Ramaraju D, Gallagher S, Hofmann M, Kim S, Zebley M, Fassler S. In-hospital and 6-month mortality rates after open elective vs open emergent colectomy in patients older than 80 years. Dis Colon Rectum. 2011;54:467–71.

74. Frasson M, Braga M, Vignali A, Zuliani W, Di Carlo V. Benefits of laparoscopic colorectal resection are more pronounced in elderly patients. Dis Colon Rectum. 2008;51:296–300.

75. Cescon M, Grazzi GL, Del Gaudio M, Ercolani G, Ravaioli M, Nardo B, Cavallari A. Outcome of right hepatectomies in patients older than 70 years. Arch Surg. 2003;138:547–52.

76. Menon KV, Al-Mukhtar A, Aldouri A, Prasad RK, Lodge PA, Toogood GJ. Outcomes after major hepatectomy in elderly patients. J Am Coll Surg. 2006;203:677–83.

77. Mazzoni G, Tocchi A, Miccini M, Betelli E, Cassini D, De Santis M, Colace L, Brozzetti S. Surgical treatment of liver metastases from colorectal cancer in elderly patients. Int J Colorectal Dis. 2007;22:77–83.

78. Figueras J, Ramos E, López-Ben S, Torras J, Albiol M, Llado L, Gonzáles HD, Rafecas A. Surgical treatment of liver metastases from colorectal cancer in elderly patients. When is it worthwhile? Clin Trans Oncol. 2007;9:392–400.

79. Di Liguori-Carino N, van Leeuwen BL, Ghaneh P, Wu A, Audisio RA, Poston GJ. Liver resection for colorectal liver metastases in older patients. Crit Rev Oncol Hematol. 2008;67:273–8.
80. Adam R, Frilling A, Elias D, Laurent C, Ramos E, Capussotti L, Poston GJ, Wicherts DA, de Haas RJ, the Liver/Met Survey Centre. Liver resection of colorectal metastases in elderly patients. Br J Surg. 2010;97:366–76.
81. Chiappa A, Makuuchi M, Lygidakis NJ, Zbar AP, Chong G, Bertani E, Sitzler PJ, Biffi R, Bianchi PP, Contino G, Misiotano P, Orsi F, Travaini L, Trifiro G, Zampino MG, Fazio N, Goldhirsch A, Andreoni B. The management of colorectal liver metastases: expanding the role of hepatic resection in the age of multimodal therapy. Crit Rev Oncol Hematol. 2009;72(1):65–75.
82. Mazzoni G, Tocchi A, Miccini M, Bettelli E, Cassin ID, De Santis M, Colace L, Brozzetti S. Surgical treatment for liver metastases from colorectal cancer in elderly patients. Int J Colorectal Dis. 2007;22:77–83.
83. Figueras J, Ramos E, Lopez-Ben S, Torres J, Albiol M, Llado L, Gonzales HD, Rafecas A. Surgical treatment of liver metastases from colorectal carcinoma in elderly patients. When is it worthwhile? Clin Transl Oncol. 2007;9:392–400.
84. Reddy SK, Barbas AS, Turley RS, Gamblin C, Geller DA, Marsh JW, Tsung A, Clary BM, Lagoo-Deenadayalan S. Major liver resection in elderly liver patients: a multi-institutional analysis. J Am Coll Surg. 2011;212:787–95.
85. Miner TJ, Jaques DP, Tavaf-Motamen H, Schriver CD. Decision making on surgical palliation based on patient outcome data. Am J Surg. 1999;177:150–4.
86. Liu SK, Church JM, Lavery IC, Fazio VW. Operation in patients with incurable colon cancer – is it worthwhile? Dis Colon Rectum. 1997;40:11–4.
87. Rosen SA, Buell JF, Yoshida A, Kazsuba S, Hurst R, Michelassi F, Millis JM, Posner MC. Initial presentation with stage IV colorectal cancer: how aggressive should we be? Arch Surg. 2000;135:530–5.
88. Wasserberg N, Kaufman HS. Palliation of colorectal cancer. Surg Oncol. 2007;16:299–310.
89. Law WL, Chan WF, Lee YM, Chu KW. Non-curative surgery for colorectal cancer: critical appraisal of outcomes. Int J Colorectal Dis. 2004;19:197–202.
90. Phang PT, MacFarlan JK, Taylor RH, Cheifetz R, Davis Nm Hay J, McGregor G, Speers C, Coldman A. Effect of emergent presentation on outcome from rectal cancer management. Am J Surg. 2003;185:450–4.
91. Ptok H, Marusch F, Steinert R, Meyer L, Lippert H, Gastinger I. Incurable stenosing colorectal carcinoma: endoscopic stent implantation or palliative surgery. World J Surg. 2006;30:1481–7.
92. Hünerbein M, Krause M, Moesta KT, Rau B, Schlag PM. Palliation of malignant rectal obstruction with self-expanding metal stents. Surgery. 2005;137:42–7.
93. Fazio VW. Indications and surgical alternatives for palliation of rectal cancer. J Gastrointest Surg. 2004;8:262–5.
94. Scheidbach H, Ptok H, Schubert D, Kose D, Hugel O, Gastinger L, Köckerling F, Lippert H. Palliative stoma creation: comparison of laparoscopic vs. conventional procedures. Langenbecks Arch Surg. 2009;394:371–4.
95. Kann BR. Early stomal complications. Clin Colon Rectal Surg. 2008;21:23–30.
96. Kimmey MB. Endoscopic methods (other than stents) for palliation of rectal carcinoma. J Gastrointest Surg. 2004;8:270–3.
97. Rao VS, Al-Mukhtar A, Rayan F, Stojkovic S, Moore PJ, Ahmad SM. Endoscopic laser ablation of advanced rectal carcinoma – DGH experience. Colorectal Dis. 2005;7:58–60.
98. Saltz LB. Palliative management of rectal cancer: the roles of chemotherapy and radiation therapy. J Gastrointest Surg. 2004;6:274–6.
99. Turler A, Schafer H, Pichlmaier H. Role of transanal endoscopic microsurgery in the palliative treatment of rectal cancer. Scand J Gastroenterol. 1997;32:58–61.
100. Michel P, Roque I, DiFiore F, Langlkois S, Scott M, Tenière P, Paillot P. Colorectal cancer with non-resectable synchronous metastases: should the primary tumor be resected? Gastroenterol Clin Biol. 2004;28:434–7.

101. Poultsides GA, Servais EL, Saltz LB, Patil S, Kemeny NE, Guillem JG, Weiser M, Temple LK, Wong WD, Paty PB. Outcome of primary tumor in patients with synchronous stage IV colorectal cancer receiving combination chemotherapy without surgery as initial treatment. J Clin Oncol. 2009;27:3379–84.
102. Tebutt NC, Norman AR, Cunningham D, Hill ME, Tait D, Oates J, Livingston S, Andreyev J. Intestinal complications after chemotherapy for patients with unresected primary colorectal cancer and synchronous metastases. Gut. 2003;52:568–73.
103. Scoggins CR, Meszoely IM, Blanke CD, Beauchamp RD, Leach SD. Nonoperative management of primary colorectal cancer in patients with stage IV disease. Ann Surg Oncol. 1999; 6:651–7.
104. Tanoue Y, Tanaka N, Nomura Y. Primary site resection is superior for incurable metastatic colorectal cancer. World J Gastroenterol. 2010;29:3561–6.
105. Soprani KM, Charachon A, Delbaldo C, Vigano L, Luciani A, Cherqui D. Primary chemotherapy with or without colonic stent for management of irresectable stage IV colorectal cancer. Eur J Surg Oncol. 2010;36:58–64.
106. Karoui M, Roudot-Thoraval F, Mesli F, Mitry E, Aparicio T, DesGuetz G, Louvet C, Landi B, Tiret E, Sobhani I. Primary colectomy in patients with stage IV colon cancer and unresectable distant metastases improves overall survival: results of a multicentric study. Dis Colon Rectum. 2011;54:930–8.
107. Ronnekliev-Kelly SM, Kennedy GD. Management of stage IV rectal cancer: palliative options. World J Gastroenterol. 2011;17:835–47.
108. Kleespies A, Fuessl KE, Seeliger H, Eichhorn ME, Muller MH, Rentsch M, Thasler WE, Angele MK, Kreis ME, Jauch KW. Determinants of morbidity and survival after elective noncurative resection of stage IV colon and rectal cancer. Int J Colorect Dis. 2009;24:1097–9.
109. Kretzschmar A, Cunningham D, Berry S. Incidence of gastrointestinal perforations and bleeding in patients starting bevacizumab treatment in first-line mCRC without primary tumour resection: preliminary results from the First BEATrial. Paper presented at American Society of Clinical Oncology gastrointestinal symposium 2006.
110. Sugrue M, Kozloff M, Hainsworth J, Badarinath S, Cohn A, Flynn P, Steis R, Dong W, Sarkar S, Grothey A. Risk factors for gastrointestinal perforations in patients with metastatic colorectal cancer receiving bevacizumab plus chemotherapy. Paper presented at American Society of Clinical Oncology 2006. J Clin Oncol 2006;24(18 Suppl; Abstr 3535).
111. Karoui M, Koubaa W, Delbaldo C, Charachon A, Laurent A, Piedbois P, Cherqui D, Tran Van Nhieu J. Chemotherapy has also an effect on primary tumor in colon carcinoma. Ann Surg Oncol. 2008;15:3440–6.
112. Seo GJ, Park JW, Yoo SB, Kim SY, Choi HS, Chang HJ, Shin A, Jeong SY, Kim DY, Oh JH. Intestinal complications after palliative treatment for asymptomatic patients with unresectable stage IV colorectal cancer. J Surg Oncol. 2010;102:94–9.
113. Costi R, Di Mauro D, Veronesi L, Ardizzoni A, Salcuni P, Roncoroni L, Sarli L, Violi V. Elective palliative resection of incurable stage IV colorectal cancer: who really benefits from it? Surg Today. 2011;41:222–9.
114. Meulenbeld HJ, Creemers G-J. First-line treatment strategies for elderly patients with metastatic colorectal cancer. Drugs Aging. 2007;24:223–38.

Chapter 8
Surgery for Liver Metastases

Nicola de' Liguori Carino and Luigi Bonanni

Abstract Life expectancy has increased significantly in recent years. Along with this even the definition of an elderly patient has been modified over the years. During the last two decades the cut-off point of 70 years became the most commonly used in literature, replacing the 65 years cut-off wider adopted in the past.

Colorectal cancer is one the most common malignant tumors in the Western world and remains the second most common cause of cancer related deaths in the United States. Up to 76% of all people affected by colorectal cancer are diagnosed between the ages of 65 and 85; and 33–50% of patients with colorectal liver metastases are 70 years old and beyond.

Over the last twenty years the number of elderly patients considered for live resection has been increasing constantly.

Nowadays, techniques in the field of hepatic surgery and peri-operative care has improved dramatically achieving mortality rates that vary between 0% and 11%, even for procedures combining colon resection with liver resection.

Recent studies published in literature showed no significant difference in postoperative complications and postoperative mortality between the age specific subgroups of patients undergoing liver resections for colorectal liver metastases. Long term survival is comparable to younger patients and a multimodality approach to metastatic disease using peri-operative chemotherapy is now established in the elderly and its use can be associated with improved results. When non resectable and only localized to the liver, colorectal liver metastases can be treated by ablative techniques such as Radiofrequency Ablation and Microwave Ablation. Such procedures, with or without the aid chemotherapy, can provide a significant improvement in overall survival.

Increasing age itself it is not a predictor of short survival therefore elderly patient affected by colorectal liver metastases should be always considered for liver resection when feasible.

N. de' Liguori Carino, M.D. (✉) • L. Bonanni, M.D.
HPB Unit, North Manchester General Hospital, Pennine Acute Trust,
Manchester M8 5RB, UK
e-mail: nicola.deliguoricarino@pat.nhs.uk

D. Papamichael, R.A. Audisio (eds.), *Management of Colorectal Cancers in Older People*,   81
DOI 10.1007/978-0-85729-984-0_8, © Springer-Verlag London 2013

Keywords Liver metastases • Colorectal metastases • Liver surgery • Colorectal • Elderly

Epidemiology and Surgical Considerations

Life expectancy has increased significantly in recent years and is now 76 years for men and 80 years for women in developed countries [1]. Along with the increase of life expectancy, even the definition of an elderly patient has been modified during the last years. During the last two decades, the cutoff point of 70 years became the most commonly used in literature, replacing the 65-year cutoff wider adopted in the past. Currently over 50 % of all malignancies are diagnosed in elderly patients. Cancer affects mainly the elderly due to a combination of lifetime exposure to carcinogens and lifestyle-related risks [2]. Moreover, the risk of cancer-related death diminishes with increasing age; it is estimated to be 40 % for those aged between 50 and 70 years, falling to 10 % for those over 90 years old [3]. Colorectal cancer is one of the most common malignant tumors in the Western world and remains the second most common cause of cancer-related deaths in the USA [4].

Worldwide about 1,200,000 new cases of colorectal cancer are diagnosed every year, and 20 % of patients have synchronous liver metastases at diagnosis [5]. Notably, after resection of primary tumor, even 20–50 % of the patients develop liver metastases in the course of their disease.

It has been reported that 76 % of all people affected by colorectal cancer are diagnosed between the ages of 65 and 85 [6, 7], and 33–50 % of patients with colorectal liver metastases (CRLMs) are 70 years old and beyond [8].

Although the prevalence of elderly colorectal cancer patients is increasing, survival in this patient category has not improved accordingly. Postoperative mortality has decreased over the past decades, but there has been no improvement in stage-specific survival rates in the elderly [9]. Despite studies showing up to 50 % of patients presenting with CRLM being elderly [10], these patients appear to be underrepresented in major series of surgical resection [11] and have been shown to be less likely to be offered surgical treatment [12]. Elderly patients are often not considered for liver resection only because of their age and were unrepresented in most clinical trials until 10 years ago. In some studies reporting resection for CRLMs, only 8–20 % of the participants were aged 70 and older [11, 13]. Over the last 20 years, the number of elderly patients considered for liver resection has been increasing constantly. Only 6 % of all patients having liver resection were aged at least 70 years in 1990; this proportion increased to 16.3 % in 2000 to 25.6 % in 2005 and 25.8 % in 2007 [14].

Age standardized survival rates are lower for elderly patients with colorectal cancer especially in the first year after diagnosis [6]. Certainly, socioeconomic factors are partly responsible for these unacceptable differences in treatment outcome. The elderly and especially those widowed or socially isolated do not seek medical help in the early stages of disease and are often not involved in screening programs. They are therefore more likely to present with stage IV disease and liver metastases.

Sadly, population-based studies have shown that age is an independent factor associated with a curative resection for CRLM [15]. It has been reported that patients over 75 years old were two to five times less likely to be offered resection of their liver metastases than younger patients. Not surprisingly, cancer-specific survival was worse in the senior group [12]. These differences suggest that, despite the evidence confirming the safety of hepatic surgery in the elderly, a large number of these patients are not referred for curative surgical treatment, probably because oncologists still have doubts about the possible benefits of liver surgery in this group of patients [16].

Such a minimalist approach would seem unacceptable as resection offers by far the best survival rates in treatment of colorectal cancer liver metastases. It is likely that concern about an expected increased postoperative morbidity and mortality in the elderly might have been a reason not to treat metastatic cancer for the past decades.

Nowadays, perioperative care has improved dramatically, and mortality rates vary between 0 and 11 %, even for procedures combining colon resection with liver resection [17]. Recent studies published in literature showed no significant difference in postoperative complications and postoperative mortality between the age-specific subgroups of patients undergoing liver resections for CRLM [4].

When patients with stage IV colorectal cancer and liver metastases receive palliative care only, mean survival rate is 4–7 months [17], while chemotherapy alone offers a progression-free survival of 7–10 months and median survival of 9–22 months only [18].

An extensive review of 30 independent studies investigating the efficacy and safety of surgical resection of colorectal liver metastases reported that approximately 30 % of patients remain alive 5 years after resection and around two-thirds of these are disease-free [19]. A recently published large series of 13.599 patients over the age of 65 diagnosed with colorectal cancer liver metastases showed that hepatectomy was associated with improved survival. Median survival was 17 months without resection and 46 months if liver resection was performed [20].

Yet, when balancing the benefits of surgical resection of liver metastases against the potential risks of surgery (i.e., complications, decrease of quality of life, and even death), many clinicians are still reluctant to advise in favor of surgical treatment in the elderly. There is an increasing need to educate and inform physicians treating elderly patients with colorectal liver metastases.

Physicians have an obligation to allow patients to enjoy the remaining years of their life in the best possible way. Offering only palliative care for liver metastases with a 0 % chance of survival in an era when safe liver resection is technically feasible is inappropriate. There are however several factors, as discussed below, to consider when selecting elderly patients for hepatic resection.

Physiological Changes in the Aging Liver

With increasing age, hepatic blood flow gradually decreases (by as much 45 %) [21], and from the age of 50 years, the size of the liver starts to decrease from 2.5 % of total body mass to roughly 1.5 % in the octogenarian [22]. The total number of hepatocytes is reduced even though the individual size of the cells may be increased which is due to an increase in biological demand. The liver function is not usually impaired in elderly patients, but synthesis of clotting factors may be reduced. The majority of hepatic functions like filtration, detoxification, ethanol elimination, and conjugation are usually not impaired in the elderly; however, when challenged, because of the decreased number of hepatocytes, hepatic synthesis of several proteins may be reduced [22]. Reduction of the hepatic acute phase response in elderly patients undergoing liver resections has been reported in literature [23].

In the younger patients, mean levels of acute phase proteins like α_1-antitrypsin and plasma fibrinogen levels increased up to 30 % after liver resection when compared to the preoperative levels, whereas in elderly patients this difference has not been reported. Acute phase proteins play an important role in the body's defense against bacterial invasion and the control of leukocyte-generated mechanisms necessary for the removal of bacteria and dead cells. The increased rate of postoperative infection found in the elderly patients was thought to be caused by the impaired acute phase response along with reduced mobility. Postoperative albumin levels and hepaplastin test values were also significantly lower in the elderly postoperatively, and prothrombin time was increased. It takes approximately 3 months in the elderly for these values to return to their normal preoperative level. Different studies have reported no difference in postoperative liver function after right hepatectomy when comparing patients aged 65 years or more to patients aged younger than 40 [24]; at the same time, no significant differences in postoperative mortality and morbidity were identified. This is in accordance with reports which showed that using donor livers from elderly patients resulted in comparable outcomes in orthotopic liver transplantation [25] Therefore, the healthy aging liver appears well able to withstand the test of surgical resection.

Liver failure is one of the most worrying postoperative complications in hepatic surgery, and it is associated with significant mortality [26, 27]. Elderly patients may be more prone to liver failure compared to younger counterparts for several reasons.

Age-related alterations of the liver may reduce the functional reserve of the organ and the tolerance to ischemic damage related to vascular clamping, often used in liver resections, which might predispose older adults to postoperative liver failure [28].

Normal hepatic parenchyma tolerates vascular exclusion for up to 45 min; in elderly patients, due to reduction in weight and blood flow, delayed regeneration, and decrease in response to certain hormones such as insulin or glucocorticoids of liver, it is possible that parenchyma ischemia may have worst effects on hepatic function. Although no conclusive data about the tolerance of the liver in aged patients to normothermic ischemia are available, presently, it is advised, whenever possible, to use portal pedicle inflow occlusion as less as possible.

Neoadjuvant Chemotherapy and Liver Surgery

The use of perioperative chemotherapy in the treatment of patients with resectable and unresectable CRLM is now well established.

In resectable CRLM, chemotherapy given in the neoadjuvant setting has the potential to reduce the overall tumor volume allowing for limited liver resections with the aim of reducing surgery-related morbidity and mortality and improving postoperative recovery [29]. It can also increase the R0 resection rate, eliminate micrometastases, and offer an in vivo biological test on tumor aggressiveness and chemosensitivity that could guide oncologist and surgeons on future treatment strategies [30].

When used with palliative intent, chemotherapy has shown to be able to achieve up to 33 % of conversion rate from initially unresectable into resectable liver lesions [29]. On the other hand, several studies have demonstrated a significant correlation among neoadjuvant chemotherapy and increase in perioperative morbidity.

In a recent paired matched analysis comparing young versus elderly patients undergoing liver resection for colorectal liver metastases, no statistical difference in terms of toxicity was observed between the two groups with no grade 3–4 hematological or nonhematological toxicities [29].

A large international multicenter cohort retrospective analysis comparing 1,624 patients over 70 years old versus 6,140 younger patients found that significantly more patients in the younger age group received preoperative chemotherapy (44.8 % vs 33.9 %) and postoperative chemotherapy (61.2 % vs 44.3 %). There was no significant survival difference between patients who did or did not have preoperative chemotherapy. In patients receiving preoperative chemotherapy, survival was inversely related to the number of cycles and lines and tended to be influenced by the response to chemotherapy. In this group of patients, a higher risk for postoperative morbidity (37.9 % vs 31.5 % for those without chemotherapy; $P=0.030$), but no difference in 60-day postoperative mortality (3.1 % vs 3.9 %; $P=0.461$), was also observed. Finally, postoperative chemotherapy emerged as an independent predictor of survival.

In a retrospective analysis of 181 consecutive liver resections for CRLM in older patients, the authors reported a rate of postoperative mortality and morbidity which was not increased in those receiving neoadjuvant chemotherapy. The use of neoadjuvant chemotherapy was found to correlate with increased overall survival, but not with disease-free survival. However, some authors suggested that results on survival analysis should have been interpreted with some care because of the relatively small numbers and short median follow-up of patients [30].

Tamandl and colleagues conducted a comparative analysis of prospectively collected data from 244 patients who underwent liver resection for CRLM. A cohort of 70 elderly patients (>70 years of age) was identified and analyzed toward possible benefits of neoadjuvant chemotherapy followed by potentially curative hepatic resection. Patients were treated either with oxaliplatin-based chemotherapy (XELOX), 5-FU alone (5-FU/LV), or no preoperative chemotherapy. In the elderly group, perioperative complication and mortality rate were similar in both groups (neoadjuvant chemotherapy vs no chemotherapy). The administration of neoadjuvant chemotherapy per se did not influence overall survival (OS) and recurrence-free survival (RFS) in all patients. However, when the neoadjuvant chemotherapy group was divided in two subgroups according to chemotherapeutic agents (XELOX and 5FU/LV) and analyzed focusing on OS and RFS, it was clear that the XELOX group benefited from this treatment achieving a significant longer RFS when compared to the 5-FU/LV and no chemotherapy groups. OS was not calculated as all patients in this group were all alive at the time of the analysis. Response to chemotherapy was the sole factor with significant prolonged RFS and survival in uni- and multivariate analyses. They concluded that the benefits of efficient combination chemotherapy and surgery with regard to longer RFS and OS outweighed the potential caveats including side effects and possible delays in the preoperative course [5].

Data from large studies suggest that neoadjuvant chemotherapy followed by hepatic resection could be performed safely in elderly patients with an acceptable rate of perioperative morbidity and mortality. Acknowledging the improvement of perioperative chemotherapy and its benefits on long-term survival, it is nowadays recommended to investigate if elderly people with colorectal liver metastases undergoing liver resection are eligible for systemic neoadjuvant chemotherapy.

Preoperative Assessment

The main potential limitation of hepatic surgery in elderly patients is the anticipated higher risk when compared to younger. Older patients are in fact more likely to present with increasing comorbidity. Associated illnesses may be the main reason why elderly patients with good functioning livers are not able to withstand the cardiovascular or pulmonary stress of major surgery. It is clear that the presence of associated medical conditions in itself is not a contraindication for major surgery. However, it is important to identify those patients that are too frail to undergo major surgery. American Society of Anesthesiology (ASA) scores can be utilized but are highly user dependent and not specific enough to predict an outcome in individual elderly patients.

Traditional exercise stress test is now more and more frequently replaced by the cardiopulmonary exercise testing (CPET) that is more often available as preoperative tool to assess individual's fitness for surgery. CPET is a noninvasive, objective method of assessing integrated responses of the heart, lungs, and musculoskeletal system to incremental exercise, which are not adequately reflected through routine measurement of individual organ system functions. It is able to provide two key indicators: the body's maximum oxygen uptake (V_ O2max) and the point at which anaerobic metabolism exceeds aerobic metabolism (ventilatory anaerobic threshold or VAT). Together, these broadly indicate the ability of the cardiovascular system to deliver oxygen to the peripheral tissues and the ability of the tissues to utilize that oxygen. It has already been demonstrated that measures such as V_ O2max are useful predictors of postoperative complications of pulmonary resection surgery and in assessing the timing of cardiac transplant surgery, while the VAT is a predictor of postoperative cardiac complications in abdominal surgery [31].

Performance status (PS) is still widely used in managing treatment options for cancer patients. The ECOG/WHO/Zubrod scale is currently the most commonly used for its simplicity. It runs from 0 to 5, with 0 denoting perfect health and 5 death. However, PS assessment can be problematic, especially in patients who have become ill quickly or where there are conflicting parameters, e.g., patients whose function is limited but who are still actively working. Moreover, many aspects of physical limitations are not totally recognized by PS, in particular those aspects of daily life that require instrumental activities (using public transportation means or the telephone) and that may affect adherence to diagnostic and treatment protocols [32].

The comprehensive geriatric assessment scale (CGA) is an instrument used by geriatricians to evaluate the condition of elderly patients and entails activities of daily living (ADL), instrumental activities of daily living (IADL), comorbidity, social support, cognitive status, and the presence of geriatric syndromes. This tool has been adapted by several investigators to predict short- and long-term mortality [33]. There are however very few tools that have been tested in the surgical setting. One CGA instrument that shows great promise in this respect is the preoperative assessment of cancer in the elderly (PACE). It has been proven to be a valuable tool in describing the functional capacity and preoperative health status in an international cohort of elderly cancer patients [34]. Preliminary data suggest that 30-day morbidity is related to IADL and the brief fatigue inventory [35]. However, no specific studies have been undertaken in the hepatobiliary setting, and its validity in this subgroup of patients remains unexplored.

Many original and review papers have now been published on liver resection for colorectal liver metastases in the elderly. All of these quote perioperative mortality and morbidities, whereas the majority of them conducted uni- and multivariate analysis to identify risk factors for poor outcome. Interestingly though, none have taken into account or analyzed preexisting comorbidities and their influence on short- and long-term results. It is then obvious that, when comparing older to young patients undergoing liver resection for colorectal liver metastases, there is a significant bias on patient selection in the elderly group. Moreover, the majority of these papers did not mention selection criteria, and none quoted the percentage of elderly patients to whom surgery was not offered due to estimated high perioperative risk. It is therefore possible that elderly patients who received surgery in all these studies did not potentially represent the average population in that age group but were a selected group with low associated comorbidities. From this observation there comes a need for a specific, reproducible, and widely adoptable preoperative tool, able to assess and stratify perioperative risks in elderly patients undergoing major cancer surgery according to preexisting associated medical conditions, enabling clinicians to have a more accurate selection of patients and allowing comparison among different studies.

Liver Resection

When possible, liver resection for CRLM remains the only treatment that can offer a chance of cure and long-term survival. Over the last decade, the combination of new chemotherapeutic agents, a better knowledge of their use and multimodality approach to stage IV colorectal cancer, has managed to improve by far the long-term survival after liver resection. More recent series have reported 5-year survival rate after hepatic resection of CRLM as high as 58 % [36]. Acknowledging the limitations of this comparison, it is a testimony to the progress that has been made.

Nowadays techniques in hepatic resection are established, and tools such as ultrasonic dissection devices, effective simultaneous cutting and coagulating devices, argon lasers, and tissue glues are now available worldwide and allow for complex open and laparoscopic liver resections. Alongside these, anesthetic interventions have been optimized in this field and dedicated perioperative pathways developed, making routine liver surgery possible and safe in large hepatobiliary units. Perioperative mortality for liver resection performed for metastatic colorectal cancer has decreased substantially over the past three decades to <5 % in most series and approximately 1 % in high-volume centers [37], whereas morbidity rate in now below 40 % [5].

Over the last few years, a number of studies have concentrated on analyzing and comparing outcomes in liver resection for CRLM in the elderly versus younger patients.

One early study reported on age as a poor prognostic factor for outcome after liver resection [38]. In later studies Brunken found that of a group of patients with liver metastases, resection was offered in 56 % of patients ≥70 years versus 68 % in the younger age group [39]. Surprisingly 5-year survival after resection was better in the elderly, but this observation was explained by the greater rate of R0 resections. This probably reflected a less advance disease stage in this group of patients which would translate into a bias of selection criteria among young and elderly patients. Despite the incidence of preoperative cardiac comorbidities being significantly higher among older patients (43 % vs 2 %), overall postoperative morbidity was comparable in both groups (28 % vs 26 %), as well as duration of hospital stay (14 vs 15 days). In a previous published series of 178 consecutive elderly patients undergoing 181 liver resections for CRLM in a single institution in a 17-year period, authors observed the median length of in-hospital stay of 13 days. Seventy (38.5 %) patients experienced postoperative complications, 27 (14.9 %) patients suffered "surgical" complications, and 43 (23.8 %) with "medical" complications. Among those who suffered complications, seven patients had transient liver failure, and three of whom (1.7 %) had fatal liver failure. Liver failure only occurred after resection of four or more liver segments; however, there was no significant difference in the postoperative complication rate among patients who underwent minor resections, compared to those who underwent major liver resections ($p=0.383$). The postoperative complication rate was not increased in those receiving neoadjuvant chemotherapy ($p=0.954$). The overall postoperative mortality rate was 4.9 %. All but one death occurred after a major resection. With a median follow-up of 17.5 months, overall and disease-free survival rates at 1, 3, and 5 years were 86.1, 43.2, and 31.5 % and 80.4, 31.6, and 17.4 %, respectively. Tumor recurred in 46.4 % of patients, where the majority of them had undergone a major liver resection (59.5 %) compared to 39.5 % of patients having undergone a minor liver resection, respectively [5].

In a previous study overlooking 25-year period matching 41 elderly versus 126 young patients undergoing liver resection for CRLM, Brand found no difference between the two groups regarding ICU stay (3.9 vs 2.0 days, respectively), length of hospital stay (13 vs 16 days), major morbidity (29 % vs 17.5 %), or mortality (7.3 % vs 2.4 %). Elderly patients tended to require more blood transfusion (46 % vs 29 %), but again this difference did not reach statistical significance. With respect to long-term outcome recurrence rate, disease-free interval and 5-year overall survival were comparable in both groups [40].

In a study by Menon et al. [27], a subgroup analysis on 126 elderly patients undergoing a major hepatectomy for colorectal liver metastases showed 3-year overall and disease-free survival to not be different from the younger group (61 % vs 55 % and 60 % vs 47 %, respectively). Zacharias evaluated short- and long-term outcome after first and repeat hepatic resection in patients older than 70 years. Results were promising but not as good as the outcomes seen in younger patients. Morbidity and mortality rates were comparable to previous series. Overall survival for patients with first liver resection was 86, 44, and 21 % at 1, 3, and 5 years, respectively. Disease-free survival was 45, 19, and 19 % at 1, 3, and 5 years, respectively. Resection of recurrent metastatic disease proved technically feasible with low morbidity and low mortality rates. One-, 2-, and 3-year survival rates were 61, 37, and 25 %, respectively, but there were no 5-year survivors after repeat resection, as disease recurred in all of them. It was concluded that repeat resection of liver metastases remains controversial [8].

All these findings coming from the above studies should be interpreted with great caution, as a selection bias is suspected in these single-center reports.

In 2010, a large multicenter retrospective analysis conducted on a total of 7,764 patients from 102 centers of 30 different countries, comparing patients of 70 years of age or older versus younger undergoing liver resection for CRLM, was published [14]. It was found that 62 (3.8 %) of 1,624 elderly patients died within 60 days from surgery, compared with 101 (1.6 %) of 6,140 in the younger group ($p<0.001$). Postoperative morbidity occurred in 32.3 % of patients aged 70 years or above and in 28.7 % of younger patients ($p<0.001$). Interestingly, the increasing age over 70 years did not impact significantly on mortality and morbidity rates. Significant difference was observed in tumor recurrence among the two groups such as 28.1 % and 35.6 % in the elderly and young group, respectively. Repeat hepatectomy for recurrent liver disease was performed in a significantly lower proportion of elderly patients than younger patients (7.6 % vs 14.1 %; $P<0.001$). Following repeat hepatectomy, postoperative mortality was zero for elderly patients and 0.2 % for the younger group.

The 3-year overall survival rate was 57.1 % in the elderly group, compared with 60.2 % in the younger group ($P<0.001$). No significant difference was found in the 3-year disease-free survival rate with 37 % in the geriatric patients and 31.9 % in the young ones ($P=0.051$). Three-year overall survival after the last resection in elderly patients who underwent a second hepatic resection was 50.9 % compared with 57.2 % after the first hepatectomy. The 3-year survival rate of older patients after the first resection did not differ with the one of younger patients who underwent more than one hepatectomy ($P=0.309$). Median survival was 57 months after the first hepatectomy for all elderly patients who had more than one hepatectomy, compared with 69 (62–76) months for the younger group. Univariate and multivariate analyses were conducted to identify factors associated with poor survival. Following multivariate analysis it emerged that the only independent prognostic factors were more than three metastases at diagnosis, bilateral metastases, concomitant extrahepatic disease, and no postoperative chemotherapy treatment. They concluded that liver resection for CRLM can offer to elderly patient an intermediate long-term survival rate with an acceptable postoperative mortality. Moreover, these results do not deteriorate with increasing age as demonstrated by patients aged 80 years or more where 3-year survival rates were comparable with those of 70–75-year-olds. In this study, postoperative mortality within

60 days of hepatectomy was indeed higher in elderly patients than in their younger counterparts. The higher perioperative mortality in the older group might be explained in part by the fact that advanced age by itself is a risk factor for higher surgical risk, although this is not related to the extent of hepatectomy. Coexisting chronic morbidity and limited survival expectancy of the elderly population were thought to be responsible for such results. They also concluded that an aggressive surgical approach should not be denied to elderly patients in light of comparable perioperative mortality rates following repeat hepatectomy among the two groups, contrasting what was previously reported in the sole publication reporting poorer outcomes for repeat hepatectomy [8].

Alternative Techniques

Unfortunately, only a minority (10–20 %) of patients affected by colorectal cancer liver metastases are candidates for curative surgery [41]. Ablative technologies, performed with a percutaneous or laparoscopic approach, in association with chemotherapy, may offer an alternative treatment for patients unfit for major abdominal surgery or general anesthesia [42].

Currently three different types of ablation technologies are available. Radiofrequency ablation (RFA) has been widely adopted for management of HCC and colorectal cancer liver metastases. This technique involves the administration of energy with a frequency of <900 kHz. Transmission of a current through tissue causes molecular friction, raising temperature and leading to cell death by coagulative necrosis [43]. Microwave ablation is currently the ablative technology preferred by most of the authors; it is based on administration of radiations between 900 MHz and 2.4 GHz causing oscillation of water molecules that generates friction resulting in coagulative necrosis [44, 45]. The technique less used is cryoablation, based on the administration of liquid nitrogen to a probe tip, causing rapid cooling of tissue and the formation of intracellular ice crystals, with disruption of tissue perfusion, leading to ischemia [43].

During the last years, the high rate of complications and the fear of cryoshock have led to cryoablation falling out of favor as the other ablative technologies demonstrated to be safer and equally effective [43].

Potential advantages of ablation techniques compared to resection include a less invasive procedure, sparing of parenchyma, and ability to perform repeated procedures. Disadvantages are inability to treat large tumors, lesions in difficult locations and in close proximity to major vascular and/or biliary structures. Peripheral lesions near the capsule should also be ablated with caution in order to avoid damage to adjacent organs [43, 44].

Ablative techniques can be delivered percutaneously or with a laparoscopic approach. Although more invasive, the surgical approach allows better visualization of the surrounding organs with possibility to protect them from heat-related injuries. Laparoscopy at the same time allows for intraoperative ultrasound, which has higher sensitivity in detection of metastatic liver deposits when compared to percutaneous procedures, offering higher chance to achieve successful treatment [45]. Although results are not comparable with liver resection, ablative techniques demonstrated improved survival rates compared to chemotherapy alone or palliative treatment.

Data reported in the literature showed overall 5-year survival rate of 33–58 % for hepatic resection and 18–46 % for percutaneous RFA [46].

One-, 3-, and 5-year survival rates after microwave ablation are, respectively, 40–91.4, 0–57, and 14–32 %. The major complication rate ranges from 0–19 %, with a minor complication rate of 6.7–90.5 %. Median survival reported is 20.5–43 months, with a local recurrence rate of 2–12.5 % [43].

Microwave ablation offers several theoretical advantages over RFA, including larger ablation volumes, shorter ablation duration, and the ability to perform multiple simultaneous ablations to increase ablation volume, as well as more predictable ablation zones around vessels [47]. However, so far no prospective trials have been conducted to directly compare microwave and radiofrequency ablation outcomes in colorectal cancer liver metastases.

Unfortunately, the existing literature on ablative techniques presents retrospective studies showing post-ablation results to be worse than liver resection; it is thus difficult to understand if these worse results obtained with ablation were mainly related to a higher number of patients affected by technically unresectable disease or multiple medical comorbidities in this group.

The precise role of ablation in the treatment algorithm for colorectal cancer liver metastases is difficult to define. Current consensus is that its use should be limited to unresectable liver lesions in absence of extrahepatic disease, resectable lesions in patients not fit for surgery, or as an adjunct to surgery, with patients having the majority of the tumor removed surgically and the remaining unresectable disease being ablated [43].

Transarterial chemoembolization (TACE) is another treatment modality available for management of unresectable hepatic colorectal metastases. Embolization of the arteries feeding the tumor results in necrosis of metastatic deposits induced by starving them of nutrients and oxygen. The secondary function of this technique is to deliver drugs in a controlled manner. These functions combine to enhance the toxic effect of the drug on the tumor while minimizing systemic side effects. Irinotecan-loaded drug-eluting beads have been shown to be safe and effective in patients with unresectable metastatic colorectal cancer. This treatment shows a significant benefit for patients who have failed first- and second-line therapy and is potentially an effective therapy when compared to the historical response rates to third- and fourth-line systemic chemotherapy [48].

Radiotherapeutic treatment modalities like selective internal radiation therapy (SIRT) have been gradually introduced over the last years and are now FDA approved for management of inoperable colorectal cancer liver metastases.

Selective internal radiation is based on injection of micron-sized embolic resin-based microspheres loaded with 90Y [49]. The treatment is based on the relative arterial hypervascularization of liver tumors [50].

The technique requires direct access to the hepatic arterial circulation, which is typically achieved by catheterization of either the femoral artery or, less commonly, the upper extremity arteries by the interventional radiologist. The antitumor effect of SIRT is related to radiation rather than embolization. If disease is present in both lobes, the whole liver can be treated during one session or during two separate sessions in which the left and right lobes are treated sequentially, with usually 30 days of separation between treatments [45]. Stubbs et al. showed a response rate of 94 % in 100 patients with colorectal liver metastases treated with SIRT followed by TACE. In 71 patients treated by the same regimen (SIRT followed by TACE), Gray et al. reported a response rate of 89 %. The latter group also found that the combination of TACE with a single injection of SIRT is considerably more effective in increasing tumor response and progression-free survival than HAC (hepatic arterial chemotherapy) alone. In addition, it has been indicated that survival is significantly longer in patients receiving systemic fluorouracil/leucovorin chemotherapy combined with SIRT than in patients treated with chemotherapy alone [50].

Conclusions

Recent evidence obtained by large single and multicentric studies showed that liver resection for colorectal liver metastases can be safely performed in elderly patients with acceptable perioperative risks. Long-term survival is comparable to younger patients, and an aggressive approach by means of repeated hepatectomy is justified by its good short- and long-term outcome. Perioperative chemotherapy is now established in all age groups, and its use can be associated with improved results.

Increasing age itself is not a predictor of short survival, and therefore patients aged 70 or above, affected by CRLM, should always be considered for liver resection whenever possible.

References

1. World Health Organisation. World Health Statistics 2009. WHO Library Cataloguing-in-Publication Data. pp. 35.
2. Franceschi S, La Vecchia C. Cancer epidemiology in the elderly. Crit Rev Oncol Hematol. 2001;39(3):219–26.
3. Ganz PA. Does (or should) chronologic age influence the choice of cancer treatment? Oncology. 1992;6(Suppl):45–9.
4. Kulik U, Framke T, Großhennig A, Ceylan A, Bektas H, Klempnauer J, Lehner F. Liver resection of colorectal liver metastases in elderly patients. World J Surg. 2011;35:2063–72.
5. de Liguori Carino N, van Leeuwen BL, Ghaneh P, Wu A, Audisio RA, Poston GJ. Liver resection for colorectal liver metastases in older patients. Crit Rev Oncol Hematol. 2008;67:273–8.
6. Quaglia A, Capocaccia R, Micheli A, Carrani E, Vercelli M. A wide difference in cancer survival between middle aged and elderly patients in Europe. Int J Cancer. 2007;120:2196–201.
7. Cooper GS, Yuan Z, Landefeld CS, Johanson JF, Rimm AA. A national population-based study of incidence of colorectal cancer and age. Implications for screening in older Americans. Cancer. 1995;75:775–81.
8. Zacharias T, Jaeck D, Oussoultzoglou E, Bachellier P, Weber JC. First and repeat resection of colorectal liver metastases in elderly patients. Ann Surg. 2004;240:858–65.

9. Mitry E, Bouvier AM, Esteve J, Faivre J. Improvement in colorectal cancer survival: a population-based study. Eur J Cancer. 2005;41(15):2297–303.

10. Bengtsson G, Carlsson G, Hafstrom L, Jönsson PE. Natural history of patients with untreated liver metastases from colorectal cancer. Am J Surg. 1981;141:586–9.

11. Fong Y, Fortner J, Sun RL, Brennan MF, Blumgart LH. Clinical score for predicting recurrence after hepatic resection for metastatic colorectal cancer: analysis of 1001 consecutive cases. Ann Surg. 1999;230:309–18.

12. Temple LK, Hsieh L, Wong WD, Saltz L, Schrag D. Use of surgery among elderly patients with stage IV colorectal cancer. J Clin Oncol. 2004;22(17):3475–84.

13. Fortner JG, Silva JS, Golbey RB, Cox EB, Maclean BJ. Multivariate analysis of a personal series of 247 consecutive patients with liver metastases from colorectal cancer. I. Treatment by hepatic resection. Ann Surg. 1984;199:306–16.

14. Adam R, Frilling A, Elias D, Laurent C, Ramos E, Capussotti L, Poston GJ, Wicherts DA, de Haas RJ. Liver resection of colorectal metastases in elderly patients. Br J Surg. 2010;97:366–76.

15. Leporrier J, Maurel J, Chiche L, Bara S, Segol P, Launoy G. A population-based study of the incidence, management and prognosis of hepatic metastases from colorectal cancer. Br J Surg. 2006;93(4):465–74.

16. Figueras J, Ramos E, López-Ben S, Torras J, Albiol M, Llado L, González HD, Rafecas A. Surgical treatment of liver metastases from colorectal carcinoma in elderly patients. When is it worthwhile? Clin Transl Oncol. 2007;9:392–400.

17. Tocchi A, Mazzoni G, Brozzetti S, Miccini M, Cassini D, Bettelli E. Hepatic resection in stage IV colorectal cancer: prognostic predictors of outcome. Int J Colorectal Dis. 2004;19(6):580–5.

18. Falcone A, Ricci S, Brunetti I, Pfanner E, Allegrini G, Barbara C, Crino L, Benedetti G, Evangelista W, Fanchini L, Cortesi E, Picone V, Vitello S, Chiara S, Granetto C, Porcile G, Fioretto L, Orlandini C, Andreuccetti M, Masi G. Phase III trial of infusional fluorouracil, leucovorin, oxaliplatin, and irinotecan (FOLFOXIRI) compared with infusional fluorouracil, leucovorin, and irinotecan (FOLFIRI) as first-line treatment for metastatic colorectal cancer: the Gruppo Oncologico Nord Ovest. J Clin Oncol. 2007;25(13):1670–6.

19. Simmonds PC, Primrose JN, Colquitt JL, Garden OJ, Poston GJ, Rees M. Surgical resection of hepatic metastases from colorectal cancer: a systematic review of published studies. Br J Cancer. 2006;94(7):982–99.

20. Cummings LC, Payes JD, Cooper GS. Survival after hepatic resection in metastatic colorectal cancer: a population-based study. Cancer. 2007;109(4):718–26.

21. Wynne HA, Cope LH, Mutch E, Rawlins MD, Woodhouse KW, James OF. The effect of age upon liver volume and apparent liver blood flow in healthy man. Hepatology. 1989;9: 297–301.

22. Aalami OO, Fang TD, Song HM, Nacamuli RP. Physiological features of aging persons. Arch Surg. 2003;138(10):1068–76.

23. Kimura F, Miyazaki M, Suwa T, Kakizaki S. Reduction of hepatic acute phase response after partial hepatectomy in elderly patients. Res Exp Med (Berl). 1996;196(5):281–90.

24. Ettorre GM, Sommacale D, Farges O, Sauvanet A, Guevara O, Belghiti J. Postoperative liver function after elective right hepatectomy in elderly patients. Br J Surg. 2001;88(1):73–6.

25. Tisone G, Manzia TM, Zazza S, De Liguori Carino N, Ciceroni C, Luca De I, Toti L, Casciani CU. Marginal donors in liver transplantation. Transplant Proc. 2004;36(3):525–6.

26. Koperna T, Kisser M, Schulz F. Hepatic resection in the elderly. World J Surg. 1998;22(4):406–12.

27. Menon KV, Al Mukhtar A, Aldouri A, Prasad RK, Lodge PA, Toogood GJ. Outcomes after major hepatectomy in elderly patients. J Am Coll Surg. 2006;203(5):677–83.

28. Di Benedetto F, Berretta M, D'Amico G, Montalti R, De Ruvo N, Cautero N, Guerrini GP, Ballarin R, Spaggiari M, Tarantino G, Di Sandro S, Pecchi A, Luppi G, Gerunda GE. Liver resection for colorectal metastases in older adults: a paired matched analysis. J Am Geriatr Soc. 2011;59:2282–90.

29. Adam R, Pascal G, Castaing D, Azoulay D, Delvart V, Paule B, Levi F, Bismuth H. Tumor progression while on chemotherapy: a contraindication to liver resection for multiple colorectal metastases? Ann Surg. 2004;240(6):1052–61.

30. Barone C, Nuzzo G, Cassano A, Basso M, Schinzari G, Giuliante F, D'Argento E, Trigila N, Astone A, Pozzo C. Final analysis of colorectal cancer patients treated with irinotecan and 5-fluorouracil plus folinic acid neo-adjuvant chemotherapy for unresectable liver metastases. Br J Cancer. 2007;97(8):1035.

31. Bhagwat M, Paramesh K. Cardio-pulmonary exercise testing: an objective approach to pre-operative assessment to define level of peri-operative care. Indian J Anaesth. 2010;54(4):286–91.

32. Repetto L, Fratino L, Audisio RA, Venturino A, Gianni W, Vercelli M, Parodi S, Dal Lago D, Gioia F, Monfardini S, Aapro MS, Serraino D, Zagonel V. Comprehensive geriatric assessment adds information to Eastern Cooperative Oncology Group performance status in elderly cancer patients: an Italian Group for Geriatric Oncology Study. J Clin Oncol. 2002;20(2):494–502.

33. Balducci L. Aging, frailty, and chemotherapy. Cancer Control. 2007;14(1):7–12.

34. Pope D, Ramesh H, Gennari R, Corsini G, Maffezzini M, Hoekstra HJ, Mobarak D, Sunouchi K, Stotter A, West C, Audisio RA. Pre-operative assessment of cancer in the elderly (PACE): a comprehensive assessment of underlying characteristics of elderly cancer patients prior to elective surgery. Surg Oncol. 2006;15(4):189–97.

35. Audisio RA, Zbar AP, Jaklitsch MT. Surgical management of oncogeriatric patients. J Clin Oncol. 2007;25(14):1924–9.

36. Choti MA, Sitzmann JV, Tiburi MF, Sumetchotimetha W, Rangsin R, Schulick RD, Lillemoe KD, Yeo CJ, Cameron JL. Trends in long-term survival following liver resection for hepatic colorectal metastases. Ann Surg. 2002;235:759–66.

37. Robertson DJ, Stukel TA, Gottlieb DJ, Sutherland JM, Fisher ES. Survival after hepatic resection of colorectal cancer metastases: a national experience. Cancer. 2009;115:752–9.

38. Gayowski TJ, Iwatsuki S, Madariaga JR, Selby R, Todo S, Irish W, Starzl TE. Experience in hepatic resection for metastatic colorectal cancer: analysis of clinical and pathologic risk factors. Surgery. 1994;116(4):703–10.

39. Brunken C, Rogiers X, Malago M, Hillert C, Zornig C, Busch C, Izbicki JR, Broelsch CE. Is resection of colorectal liver metastases still justified in very elderly patients? Chirurg. 1998;69(12):1334–9.

40. Brand MI, Saclarides TJ, Dobson HD, Millikan KW. Liver resection for colorectal cancer: liver metastases in the aged. Am Surg. 2000;66(4):412–5.

41. Adam R, Vinet E. Regional treatment of metastasis: surgery of colorectal liver metastases. Ann Oncol. 2004;15 Suppl 4:iv103–6.

42. Sato M, Watanabe Y, Kashu Y, Nakata T, Hamada Y, Kawachi K. Sequential percutaneous microwave coagulation therapy for liver tumor. Am J Surg. 1998;175:322–4.

43. Pathak S, Jones R, Tang JMF, Parmar C, Fenwick S, Malik H, Poston G. Ablative therapies for colorectal liver metastases: a systematic review. Colorectal Dis. 2011;13:252–65.

44. Rocha FG, D'Angelica M. Treatment of liver colorectal metastases: role of laparoscopy, radiofrequency ablation, and microwave coagulation. J Surg Oncol. 2010;102:968–74.

45. Scott DJ, Fleming JB, Watumull LM, Lindberg G, Tesfay ST, Jones DB. The effect of hepatic inflow occlusion on laparoscopic radiofrequency ablation using simulated tumors. Surg Endosc. 2002;16:1286–91.

46. Fegiz G, Ramacciato G, D'Angelo F, Barillari P, Indinnimeo M, Gozzo P, Aurello P, Valabrega S, De Angelis R. Patient selection and factors affecting results following resection for hepatic metastases from colorectal carcinoma. Int Surg. 1991;76:58–63.

47. Izzo F. Other thermal ablation techniques: microwave and interstitial laser ablation of liver tumors. Ann Surg Oncol. 2003;10:491–7.

48. Martin RC, Robbins K, Tomalty D, O'Hara R, Bosnjakovic P, Padr R, Rocek M, Slauf F, Scupchenko A, Tatum C. Transarterial chemoembolisation (TACE) using irinotecan-loaded beads for the treatment of unresectable metastases to the liver in patients with colorectal cancer: an interim report. World J Surg Oncol. 2009;7:80.

49. Prompers L, Bucerius J, Brans B, Temur Y, Berger L, Felix M. Mottaghy selective internal radiation therapy (SIRT) in primary or secondary liver cancer. Methods. 2011;55:253–7.

50. Welsh J, Kennedy A. Selective internal radiation therapy for liver metastases secondary to colorectal adenocarcinoma. Int J Radiat Oncol Biol Phys. 2006;66(2 Suppl):S62–73.

Chapter 9
Rectal Cancer Radiotherapy and Older Patients: Evidence-Based or Opinion-Based Treatment?

Rob Glynne-Jones and Kannon Nathan

Abstract Colorectal cancer is the most common malignancy in patients aged 75 years or older, and the incidence is likely to rise further as the population ages and survival increases. Sound data on the adherence to guidelines for the elderly and the uptake of treatment in the elderly is limited. However, the evidence available suggests that clinical attitudes observed regarding age and cancer treatment are consistent, such that older people with colorectal cancer tend to be offered less intensive treatment or no treatment. So how do doctors balance chronological age, comorbidity and social isolation, and other influences on their clinical decision making?

Keywords Colorectal cancer • Chemotherapy • Radiotherapy • Toxicity • Compliance • Decision making

Introduction

Colorectal cancer is the second commonest cause of cancer-related death in western countries, affects men and women almost equally, and is the most common malignancy in patients aged 75 years or older [1, 2]. As the population ages and survival increases, the incidence of rectal cancer will rise. Each year approximately 15,000 patients in the UK develop rectal cancer, which is a major cause of morbidity and mortality in the elderly. Approximately 50 % are over 70 years of age, and 20 % are

R. Glynne-Jones, FRCP, FRCR (✉)
Clinical Oncology, Mount Vernon Cancer Centre,
Rickmansworth Road, Northwood, Middlesex HA6 2RN, UK
e-mail: rob.glynnejones@nhs.net

K. Nathan, MRCP, FRCR, B.Sc.
Clinical Oncology, Mount Vernon Cancer Centre,
Middlesex HA6 2RN, UK

D. Papamichael, R.A. Audisio (eds.), *Management of Colorectal Cancers in Older People*, 95
DOI 10.1007/978-0-85729-984-0_9, © Springer-Verlag London 2013

over 80 years [3]. Recent guidelines recognize that treatment of very elderly patients is going to become an increasingly common issue because of increased life expectancy across Europe [4], but data on the adherence to guidelines for the elderly and the uptake of preoperative radiotherapy in rectal cancer in the elderly is limited.

In defining the elderly, we have set the cutoff age of 70 years as the threshold conventionally chosen by the scientific community to define old age, and it is also the indicator most widely used in reports of treatment. Population data suggests that the life expectancy of the average 70-year-old woman is 16 years and a 70-year-old man is 13 years, and the average 80-year-old has a life expectancy of 9 and 7 years, respectively [5]. The significance of age as an individual prognostic factor is topical and remains controversial.

In some studies, long-term colorectal cancer-related outcomes appear similar in the elderly to the outcomes in younger patients [6, 7]. In contrast, studies from large registries have used multivariate analysis, to show that age >70, comorbidity, and having two or more complications all had a highly significant negative effect on survival [8] – despite adjusting for other prognostic factors. In the SEER data older patients have lower cancer-specific survival than younger patients [9] – particularly in the >70 year olds (HR 1.37, CI 1.33–1.42 $p < 0.0001$), which relates mainly to the low use of radiotherapy in stage III patients. Even after more conservative surgical procedures such as local excision instead of radical surgery, elderly patients are less likely to receive radiation [9].

Traditionally, there has been a high local recurrence rate in rectal cancer. The evidence from modern-randomized trials suggests that in resectable rectal cancers, short-course preoperative radiotherapy (SCPRT) and preoperative chemoradiation (CRT) followed by total mesorectal excision (TME) have reduced the risk of local *recurrence* [10–16] to below 10 % and are routinely delivered in fit younger patients. Preoperative treatment confers an increased risk of surgical complications including a 2–8 % postoperative death rate [17, 18] which may reach 30 % at 6 months in those over 85 years [19] and a long-term impact on anorectal, urinary, and sexual function [20, 21]. Deterioration in bowel function is common following anterior resection and is more pronounced in the elderly. In addition, patients with low cancers may require a permanent stoma, which can be associated with high psychological morbidity and be more difficult for the elderly to manage. Severe comorbidity is also a competing risk which may also shorten life expectancy and outweigh potential gains from adjuvant radiotherapy.

More locally advanced and unresectable rectal cancers may present with bleeding, pain on defecation or pain in the distribution of the sciatic nerve, a copious mucous discharge, infections, and rarely obstruction and sets problems in management even for younger patients. Older people may also ignore or accept symptoms such as incontinence and a change in bowel habit and present with more advanced disease.

In rectal cancer improvements such as a reduction in local recurrence – when examined from the aspect of population data – have been mainly confined to younger patients [19]. In the over 85-year-old patient, 31-day mortality is 10–15 %, but 6-month mortality is in the region of 30 % [19]. Although surgical mortality is the main consideration in deciding between surgery and radiotherapy for the elderly, in our decision making we should therefore take into account the potential for local recurrence, survival, surgical morbidity, and functional outcomes – albeit from the perspective of the elderly.

Many studies find high levels of cardiovascular disease, diabetes mellitus, respiratory disease, and renal insufficiency in the elderly. Hence, the elderly are expected to experience more comorbidity, and oncologists have concerns regarding the tolerability and acceptability of radiotherapy in elderly populations over 80 years. Partly this reflects the increased comorbidity in this age group where rectal cancer becomes increasingly common [19]. However, the relevance of age "per se" to determine treatment pathways has been controversial.

Late functional effects may also be worse because of the aging effects on function of the anal sphincter (a degree of incontinence may already be present). Yet other problems such as impotence may be less relevant to some individuals because of the accepted aging effects on libido and sexual performance. In contrast, we probably do not need to be so concerned with the risk of second malignancies in an aging population.

Pooled analyses confirm that 5FU-based palliative and adjuvant chemotherapy in colon cancer offers similar efficacy to fit elderly patients as younger individuals, although there is controversy as to the additional benefit of oxaliplatin in the adjuvant setting. It is assumed that chemotherapy has similar efficacy in rectal cancer but does age itself impact on the risk of cancer recurrence in rectal cancer as in breast cancer [22].

Balancing the interplay between efficacy, comorbidity, the side effects of treatment, and cancer outcomes at any age is difficult. Even when we have a clear understanding ourselves as oncologists, we are unskilled at explaining the risk-benefit of treatment. Indeed we do not always explain the appropriate and relevant information to the elderly [23].

Several population-based [6, 9, 24–27] and retrospective studies [28] suggest that elderly patients with colorectal cancer are undertreated with substandard treatments. Treatment of rectal cancer is clearly influenced by patient's age. In the Swedish Rectal Cancer Registry, older patients ≥75 years received preoperative radiotherapy less often than younger patients regardless of surgical technique – overall 34 % versus 67 % $p < 0.001$. In a more recent population-based study [29], only 59.0 % of patients ≥75 years with rectal cancer received adjuvant radiotherapy versus 85.3 % of those younger than 75 ($p < .001$), not entirely explained by the presence of comorbidity.

Although there is little evidence-based guidance for radiotherapy and chemoradiotherapy decisions in the elderly, radiation oncologists appear to have more concerns regarding the tolerability and acceptability of radiotherapy in elderly populations, particularly in patients over 80 years, who make up approximately 25 % of our MDT discussions in the UK. Oncologists acknowledge that such patients are likely to survive 5 years despite comorbidity, and that radical treatments are effective. Yet, concerns regarding the acute toxicity and tolerability of both radiotherapy and chemoradiation (especially in those who are less fit than those eligible for clinical trials) and a systematic failure to consider elderly patients as suitable for treatment

have led to undertreatment of this age group. This bias may reflect data from historical trials which show more pronounced side effects in older patients, e.g., the
Stockholm I and II trials [30] although modern high-precision radiotherapy is much
better tolerated than parallel-opposed techniques used in these previous trials.

This chapter reviews the issues regarding radiotherapy and 5FU-based chemoradiation in elderly patients with rectal cancer. We review recent reports regarding
radiotherapy treatment in the elderly. We discuss the selection of patients who are
appropriate for preoperative chemoradiotherapy (CRT) and short-course preoperative radiotherapy (SCPRT), and the selection of patients unfit for radical surgery
who may be suitable for radical radiotherapy. We describe the various available
doses fractionation schemes and techniques and examine more palliative treatments.
Finally we recommend specific studies to accumulate evidence for decision making
and define the optimal way to treat elderly patients with rectal cancer.

The Evidence from Prospective Randomized Clinical Trials

Randomized trials in rectal cancer have provided little information on specific toxicity
and efficacy outcomes in the elderly. A pooled analysis of nine randomized EORTC
trials suggests that elderly patients fit enough to be eligible for clinical trials probably
derive a similar benefit from pelvic radiation treatment [31] with similar toxicity as
younger patients, although survival was worse for the older group of patients >70 years
with rectal cancer ($p=0.04$). In the subgroup of patients with rectal cancer, with doses
ranging between 34.5 Gy in 15 fractions and 46–50 Gy in 25 fractions, the report
detailed acceptable toxicity (12 % rectal complications and 10 % urinary dysfunction). So should elderly patients be treated exactly the same as younger patients provided there is no significant comorbidity? Clinical trials could potentially answer this
problem by ensuring that similar populations receive different treatments. However,
there has been long-standing concern regarding how representative such patients
within the trials are, when compared to the background population [32], and to what
extent the results of clinical trials can be generalized to the population seen in routine
care. It is well accepted that historically, there has been a major discrepancy in enrolment of the elderly within clinical trials [33, 34]. In the absence of direct evidence, we
are reliant on pooled analyses and metanalyses [35, 36].

Clinical trials run the risk of setting restrictive entry criteria which tend even if
not limited by eligibility to result in a population that is younger and fitter than that
seen in routine practice. While this may be justified in terms of safety and trial
administration, the net result can be a set of clinical trials whose populations are
substantially different from the population seen in practice.

Trials have mostly included fit elderly patients fulfilling specific inclusion criteria. A number of the randomized phase III trials have imposed eligibility upper age
limits <75 years or <80 years [13–15, 37, 38].

Two large randomized trials have each reported that in resectable cancers, SCPRT
and CRT are equivalent in terms of outcomes such as local recurrence, disease-free

survival (DFS), overall survival (OS), and toxicity [21, 39]. In the UK, SCPRT is increasingly being used with an interval to surgery or as a radical treatment ± brachytherapy. SCPRT is considered to have the advantage of rapid delivery and high compliance for patients who are frail, elderly, and with cardiac and renal comorbidities which preclude 5FU-based chemotherapy.

The interim results of the Stockholm III trial randomize between three arms: SCPRT proceeding to immediate surgery within a week, SCPRT and delayed surgery after 4–8 weeks, and 50 Gy in 25 fractions with surgery after a similar interval [40]. Early pathological endpoints, feasibility, compliance, and complications after RT and surgery in the initial 303 patients, suggest that SCPRT is effective with a 12 % pathological complete response rate in patients who proceeded to SCPRT and surgery after an interval of 4–8 weeks. Two small retrospective studies [41, 42] report similar tolerability and efficacy of SCPRT with an interval to allow tumor response.

Further long-term studies aimed at this specific patient population using well-established geriatric endpoints are required to clarify issues surrounding acute and late toxicity, HQOL, and functional sequelae from radiotherapy.

The Evidence from Retrospective Nonrandomized Studies

There are at least 15 population-based studies which examine the relevance of age to management of rectal cancer [6, 9, 19, 24–27, 43–50]. Most reported higher short-term mortality rates than small retrospective series or cohort studies, and all show a low uptake in radiotherapy. They suggest that elderly patients with colorectal cancer may be undertreated with nonstandard treatments.

Individual retrospective studies generally have included small numbers and are rarely homogeneous as to the populations included. Information is often lacking in terms of radiotherapy field size and doses received, interruptions and dose modifications, and the precise delivery of chemotherapy used (prolonged venous infusion, bolus 5FU, or capecitabine/UFT). In addition, the heterogeneity of multiple radiation oncologists performing or supervising CRT for the majority of patients blurs the utility of the information. The tolerability of preoperative radiotherapy appeared to be similar whether fit or with mild comorbidity, suggesting that elderly patients with rectal cancer with mild comorbidities could probably receive the same treatment as fit elderly patients.

Several retrospective studies recommend patients with resectable rectal cancer, irrespective of age, should receive preoperative radiotherapy to avoid local recurrence, and that treatment is tolerated no differently to younger patients [3, 51].

Acute Toxicity

Expected acute side effects include nausea, vomiting, diarrhea, proctitis, tenesmus, urinary frequency and dysuria, erythema, and moist desquamation of the perineum in low rectal cancers. There is a lack of good quality-specific data concerning acute complications related with adjuvant radiotherapy in the elderly – particularly those with some degree of comorbidity. Part of the problem is that there is no widely accepted comorbidity scale that has been used in studies to group and analyze such patients, so we cannot compare like with like. Gender and body mass index may provide better potential markers of acute toxicity than age in fit elderly patients [52]. In turn because women live longer than men, women will predominate in studies of the very elderly. Many studies suggest that older patients experience similar toxicity with radiotherapy and chemoradiotherapy to younger patients with acceptable compliance and hence should be treated (if fit) no different to younger patients [51, 53–55]. Other more recent studies are less positive. A recent study showed 36 patients aged 75 years or older [56] who received treatment for rectal cancer – 21 (58 %) preoperative chemoradiotherapy and 12 patients (33 %) postoperative chemoradiation [56]. Despite the fact that these patients were deemed fit enough for chemoradiation and 86 % had ECOG PS 0 or 1, the majority of patients (30/36) experienced at least one deviation from the intended treatment course, i.e., 9 (25 %) required an RT treatment break of 1–133 days, 3 (8 %) failed to receive the original planned RT dose, and in 12 (33 %) chemotherapy was dose reduced, interrupted, or discontinued.

Oral capecitabine has been recommended in the elderly because it reduces the frequency of a toxicities compared with bolus 5-FU, including stomatitis, which can be particularly debilitating in elderly patients [5]. However, capecitabine despite also its convenience may not be the ideal partner in a chemoradiation schedule for elderly patients. The MRC FOCUS 2 study [57] was designed to study efficacy and tolerability of chemotherapy for colorectal cancer in the elderly and frail not considered suitable for standard chemotherapy. With a median age of 74 and a total of 459 patients, the results show that all cause ≥G3 acute toxicity was 27 % for 5FU and 37 % for single agent capecitabine. Capecitabine is a common partner in chemoradiation in the UK.

Late Toxicity

Late long-term adverse effects of SCPRT and TME surgery on functional outcome are considerable [58], although the elderly patient may not survive long enough to express fully the late effects of radiation. Some studies suggest a relationship between more severe grades of comorbidity and the risk of late complications [55]. It is vital that clinicians take a range of characteristics into account when recommending any radical treatment approach if we are to balance the significant benefits and negative impact which can be caused.

Functional Outcomes

The poor functional outcome of rectal cancer treatment is a recognized major problem after surgery and radiotherapy, particularly in the elderly. Gastrointestinal (GI) symptoms are a common sequelae of pelvic radiotherapy and have a major impact on quality of life [59–61]. Incontinence problems in particular lead to avoidance of certain activities, such as long-distance travel by car or plane because of poor access to toilet facilities [62]. Bowel and urinary dysfunction can have a negative impact on a patient's physical, psychological, social, and emotional functioning, as well as the patient's overall well-being. Since many of these side effects, e.g., mucus leakage, flatulence, fecal incontinence, diarrhea, and constipation, increase in frequency along with aging, the elderly may be more susceptible to such problems.

Second Malignancies

High-dose radiotherapy to the pelvis increases the risk of second primary cancers, particularly for cancers of the colon, rectum, bladder, and leukemia, but the latency period for solid tumors is long. Hence, the risk of second malignancies from radiotherapy can probably be ignored in the elderly as the lag time is in the region of 10 years before this risk becomes observed, and this time frame may be even longer for brachytherapy [63].

HQOL: Health-Related Quality of Life

There are few reports of the impact of adjuvant treatments on HRQoL in elderly patients, but there is little to suggest that HRQOL is worse in the >75 age group than younger patients [64].

Chemotherapy

For chemotherapy, concerns regarding toxicity and tolerability of treatment mean that elderly patients are often underrepresented in clinical trials – receiving less aggressive combined treatments and less invasive interventions. In a recent FFCD trial of FOLFOX and FOLFIRI in colorectal cancer [65], multivariate analysis both performance status and age were independent predictors for hematologic toxicity ($p = .01$ and $p = .008$, respectively). Findings from the ACCENT database of six clinical trials suggest that adjuvant oxaliplatin-based therapies may be less effective for the elderly than for younger patients, but other biases may be present, and other patient characteristics more relevant to outcome than age. Although patients across Europe have a median age at presentation of 71 years, only 20 % of patients recruited to large-scale randomized trials chemotherapy are aged 70 years or older, which makes it difficult to extrapolate these results to help plan the treatment of elderly patients with rectal cancer – particularly when they have added comorbidities. Extrapolation of the results to patients with comorbidities is even more uncertain because the majority of patients included in the trials had only mild or no comorbidities.

There are also competing risks which impact on the endpoint of overall survival. More than three clinically significant comorbidities can determine a short life expectancy of 5 years or less. It should also be recognized that disabilities leading to difficulty in performing daily tasks and other geriatric syndromes, such as dementia, delirium and falls, may all impact on survival and probably should be given greater weight when making clinical decisions. In addition, a recent consensus meeting on colorectal cancer in the UK, during an audience debate about treatment regimens for the elderly, there was general agreement that patient choice is also key.

In the future with pharmacogenomics, we may be better placed to predict toxicity, since common gene polymorphisms may influence the toxicity of chemotherapy agents. In a recent study multivariate analysis showed a GSTP1 Ile105Val polymorphism ($p=0.041$) was the only factor found to be associated with hematological toxicity in the elderly [66].

Fractionation/Radiation Schedules

There is a widely held belief that the elderly tolerate radiotherapy less well than younger patients and require short hypofractionated regimens of radiotherapy. Although compliance may be higher, there will be a greater risk of late toxicity.

Brachytherapy

In terms of radiotherapy, there may be a role for a more conformal approach using brachytherapy either used alone, i.e., without pelvic external beam radiotherapy or in combination with external beam radiotherapy or chemoradiotherapy as an alternative radical treatment. This technique is quick, simple, and acceptable to the elderly. High-dose rate intraluminal brachytherapy (HDR-ILBT) has the advantage of high conformality – i.e., a rapid falloff of radiation dose, which allows the delivery of a high dose to the tumor while sparing normal surrounding structures such as the anal sphincter, bladder, urethra, and small bowel [67]. This strategy could be advantageous in reducing both acute and late toxicity while optimizing local tumor response and symptom control and compares favorably with IMRT. However, there is limited data available evaluating the advantages of HDR-ILBT with EBRT as compared to EBRT/CRT [68]. HDR-ILBT has been used both palliatively and to dose escalate after chemoradiation for curative treatment [69, 70]. A recent study suggest that CRT and brachytherapy offer an alternative to radical surgery in the elderly since integrating HDR-ILBT is easy and may be more effective than EBRT alone [71]. Patients treated with HDR-ILBT in addition to external beam radiation achieved a complete pathological response (pCR) rate of 58.8 % compared to 15.8 % in patients who were treated with external beam radiation alone [71]. Our own departments experience of 79 patients treated 2001–2007 with HDR-ILBT using a single line source 2-cm-diameter rectal applicator has also shown encouraging tumor and symptom response rates and acceptable toxicity [70].

Assessment

To select and deliver the most appropriate treatment, a good collaboration between surgeons, clinical nurse specialists, and radiation oncologists is necessary. In the UK, this approach is facilitated by the multidisciplinary team meeting (MDT), which is intended to discuss every patient.

It is a widely held belief that chronological age (the length of time a person has been alive) and biological age (the physical condition of their individual organs) may in some individuals be very different and that doctors should take more account of biological age. Most oncologists at least pay lip service to this principal, but estimates of the patients' ability to tolerate the acute side effects are the most important factor in decision making, and chronological age is clearly used as a measure of fitness to receive treatment.

Traditionally to determine suitability for treatment, patients were assessed for chemotherapy and radiotherapy using ECOG performance status and Karnofsky performance status, together with blood tests such as renal and liver function tests. Blood tests can reveal biochemical markers of frailty such as a low albumin, cholesterol, and hemoglobin [72]. However, these assessments do not take into account comorbidity, which the Charlson comorbidity index (CCI) can provide [73]. The ability to complete activities of daily living and instrumental activities of daily living have been shown to predict the risk of toxicity from chemotherapy and treatment-related morbidity and mortality [74].

Hence, the CCI provides a score based on common comorbidities to provide both a reliable marker of progression-free survival and mortality in the elderly cancer patient [75, 76]. A recent study of chemoradiotherapy in elderly patients highlighted that comorbidity alone cannot be used to assess patients and that individual functionality is important [56].

The International Society for Geriatric Oncology advocates a comprehensive geriatric assessment (CGA) tool to identify baseline factors which can influence treatment tolerability and guide the decision making process. The CGA not only evaluates patient comorbidity but also assesses psychological status, social support, cognition, and functional status. It is a detailed tool encompassing nutrition, polypharmacy, psychological baseline, functional needs of ADLs and IADLs, comorbidity, cognitive status, social support, and psychological status [74]. The tool however needs the expertise of a multidisciplinary team and be quite time-consuming and cumbersome to perform on each and every elderly patient.

The vulnerable elders survey-13 (VES-13) is an abbreviated CGA, which can be used as an effective screening tool. VES-13 is a self-survey of 13 items covering age, function, and comorbidities and can take less than 5 min to complete [77]. A score of ≥3 identifies as patients a vulnerable and at higher risk of functional decline during 2 years compared to scores less than 3. Therefore, patients scoring greater than 3 should be further assessed with a CGA [79]. VES-13 had been effectively used in prostate cancer assessment [78]. Using suggestions from Rodin and Mohile [79], a proposed framework for rectal cancer could be adopted.

All patients >65 years should do a VES-13. If score <3, then treat as normal. If score ≥3, then the patient should undergo a CGA. If CGA negative, then dose modify treatment accordingly and consider even short-course radical treatments where appropriate. If CGA positive, then the patient could be deemed as frail and would not tolerate potential treatment toxicities and should be managed with supportive care.

Discussion

In conclusion, patients in the West with rectal cancer are often elderly with significant comorbidities and poor social support. Since the majority of rectal cancers occur in older people and with the knowledge that we have an increasingly elderly population, it is important to optimize the most appropriate treatment strategies among this subgroup of the population, which may be different to younger cohorts. For this reason, we believe the evidence presented in this chapter demonstrates that if we are to get the risk-benefit ratio of treatment right for elderly patients, individualization of treatment by means of a comprehensive geriatric assessment is of critical importance. Chronological age "per se" should not influence our decisions. We also recommend patients should be assessed in a multidisciplinary fashion at least once weekly during radiotherapy with regard to toxicity and their overall tolerance to treatment. It is important to maximize patient tolerance with the use of simple antiemetics, antidiarrheals, analgesia, and nutritional support.

The evidence we have suggests that elderly patients with rectal cancer run the risk of both under and overtreatment with regard to external beam radiotherapy. There is a delicate balance between toxicity and survival, which is clearly different to younger patients. At the age of 80, life expectancy for a reasonably active woman is 9 years and 7 years for a man, so decisions are probably based more on our estimation of tolerability and side effects, than the benefits in terms of tumor control and survival. However, it is unclear how doctors balance chronological age, comorbidity and social isolation, and other potentially relevant influences on their clinical decision making. Do we make the same assessments and use similar patterns across all different types of cancer and the various stages of cancer as we do in younger individuals? Finally, are there differences in these approaches to the treatment of the elderly in different countries? Do the decisions depend on the age of the clinician making the decision?

The optimal treatment strategy in terms of radiotherapy and surgery for this group of patients has not been adequately defined. Population-based studies offer substantial information, but cannot capture all the data needed. It is possible that in an aging population a significant number of patients have already received radiotherapy for prostate, bladder, or gynecological cancers. Also it is not possible to identify why doctors choose not to offer or to discontinue adjuvant treatment for elderly patients or what proportion of patients themselves either decline to start or continue further treatment. Randomized studies have not specifically addressed this issue. In retrospective studies, worsening of the patient's performance status appears to be the most common reason for stopping, suggesting elderly patients may be more susceptible to experience treatment-related fatigue and debility. A systematic review of the evidence on the efficacy and particularly tolerability of cancer treatment in the over 70s and especially in the over 80s would be helpful. A table of all the relevant G3/4 toxicities in patients according to their decade, i.e., sexagenarians to nonagenarians – alongside their performance status and geriatric assessment and life expectancy would be a useful aide-memoire for clinicians. After all, we have comparisons in randomized trials for each arm.

To overcome our individual biases and select and deliver the most appropriate treatment, a good collaboration between surgeons clinical nurse specialists and radiation oncologists is necessary. In the UK, this approach is facilitated by the multidisciplinary team meeting (MDT), which is intended to discuss every patient. Better selection and a refocusing on risk-benefit of pelvic radiotherapy and radical surgery is urgently required. Improvements in the accuracy and delivery of radiotherapy may allow EBR/CRT and HDR-ILBT as an alternative local treatment in both the radical and palliative setting. In the future there could be more complex conformal radical alternatives, but as yet there are no widely accepted effective schedules or doses in common use across Europe. The simplest and most effective way to provide information is to promote a specifically designed radiotherapy rectal trial for the elderly. The MRC FOCUS 2 study [57] by recruiting 459 patients well ahead of target demonstrates that it is possible to perform randomized trials specifically in the elderly and frail.

It is therefore a priority to develop guidelines to support medical and radiation oncologists in evaluating clinical characteristics and recommending the most appropriate treatments to elderly patients. Patients also need to be part of the decision – which they are clearly not at the present time – so there needs to be tailored information in an acceptable format, aimed at supporting older people who are either considering or undergoing treatment. Checklists to ensure that we offer the relevant and appropriate information may be helpful. To drive this initiative forward, the UK example of NICE in setting breast cancer quality standards (which currently includes active treatment rates for older people) may need to be extended to cancer quality standards for colorectal/rectal cancer.

References

1. Boyle P, Langman JS. ABC of colorectal cancer: epidemiology. BMJ. 2000;321(7264):805–8.
2. Boyle P, Leon ME. Epidemiology of colorectal cancer. Br Med Bull. 2002;64:1–25. Review.
3. Martijn H, Vulto JC. Should radiotherapy be avoided or delivered differently in elderly patients with rectal cancer? Eur J Cancer. 2007;43(15):2301–6.
4. Papamichael D, Audisio R, Horiot JC, et al. Treatment of the elderly colorectal cancerpatient: SIOG expert recommendations. Ann Oncol. 2009;20(1):5–16.

5. Lichtman SM. Management of advanced colorectal cancer in older patients. Oncology (Williston Park). 2005;19(5):597–602.

6. Endreseth BH, Romundstad P, Myrvold HE, Bjerkeset T, Wibe A, Norwegian Rectal Cancer Group. Rectal cancer treatment of the elderly. Colorectal Dis. 2006;8(6):471–9.

7. Devon KM, Vergara-Fernandez O, Victor JC, McLeod RS. Colorectal cancer surgery in elderly patients: presentation, treatment, and outcomes. Dis Colon Rectum. 2009;52(7):1272–7.

8. Shahir MA, Lemmens VE, van de Poll-Franse LV, Voogd AC, Martijn H, Janssen-Heijnen ML. Elderly patients with rectal cancer have a higher risk of treatment-related complications and a poorer prognosis than younger patients: a population-based study. Eur J Cancer. 2006;42(17):3015–21.

9. Chang GJ, Skibber JM, Feig BW, Rodriguez-Bigas M. Are we undertreating rectal cancer in the elderly? An epidemiologic study. Ann Surg. 2007;246(2):215–21.

10. Peeters KC, Marijnen CA, Nagtegaal ID, Kranenbarg EK, Putter H, Wiggers T, Dutch Colorectal Cancer Group, et al. The TME trial after a median follow-up of 6 years: increased local control but no survival benefit in irradiated patients with resectable rectal carcinoma. Ann Surg. 2007;246(5):693–701.

11. Sebag-Montefiore D, Stephens RJ, Steele R, Monson J, Grieve R, Khanna S, et al. Preoperative radiotherapy versus selective postoperative chemoradiotherapy in patients with rectal cancer (MRC CR07 and NCIC-CTG C016): a multicentre, randomized trial. Lancet. 2009;373(9666):811–20.

12. van Gijn W, Marijnen CA, Nagtegaal ID, Kranenbarg EM, Putter H, Wiggers T, Dutch Colorectal Cancer Group, et al. Preoperative radiotherapy combined with total mesorectal excision for resectable rectal cancer: 12-year follow-up of the multicentre, randomized controlled TME trial. Lancet Oncol. 2011;12(6):575–82.

13. Sauer R, Becker H, Hohenberger W, Rodel C, Wittekind C, Fietkau R, German Rectal Cancer Study Group, et al. Preoperative versus postoperative chemoradiotherapy for rectal cancer. N Engl J Med. 2004;351:1731–40.

14. Bosset JF, Collette L, Calais G, Mineur L, Maingon P, Radosevic-Jelic L, et al. Chemoradiotherapy with preoperative radiotherapy in rectal cancer. N Engl J Med. 2006;355:1114–23.

15. Gerard JP, Conroy T, Bonnetain F, Bouche O, Chapet O, Closon-Dejardin MT, et al. Preoperative radiotherapy with or without concurrent fluorouracil and leucovorin in T3-T4 rectal cancers: results of FFCD 9203. J Clin Oncol. 2006;24:4620–5.

16. Roh MS, Colangelo LH, O'Connell MJ, Yothers G, Deutsch M, Alegra CJ, et al. Preoperative multimodality therapy improves disease-free survival in patients with carcinoma of the rectum: NSABP R03. J Clin Oncol. 2009;27:5124–30.

17. Paun BC, Cassie S, MacLean AR, Dixon E, Buie WD. Postoperative complications following surgery for rectal cancer. Ann Surg. 2010;251(5):807–18.

18. Borowski DW, Bradburn DM, Mills SJ, Bharathan B, Wilson RG, Ratcliffe AA, Kelly SB. Volume-outcome analysis of colorectal cancer-related outcomes. Br J Surg. 2010;97:1416–30.

19. Rutten HJ, den Dulk M, Lemmens VE, van de Velde CJ, Marijnen CA. Controversies of total mesorectal excision for rectal cancer in elderly patients. Lancet Oncol. 2008;9(5):494–501.

20. Gervaz PA, Wexner SD, Pemberton JH. Pelvic radiation and anorectal function: introducing the concept of sphincter-preserving radiation therapy. J Am Coll Surg. 2002;195:387–94.

21. Bujko K, Nowacki MP, Nasierowska-Guttmejer A, for the Polish Colorectal Study Group. Long-term results of a randomized trial comparing preoperative short-course radiotherapy with preoperative conventionally fractionated chemoradiation for rectal cancer. Br J Surg. 2006;93(10):1215–23.

22. Ring A, Sestak I, Baum M, Howell A, Buzdar A, Dowsett M, Forbes JF, Cuzick J. Influence of comorbidities and age on risk of death without recurrence: a retrospective analysis of the Arimidex, Tamoxifen alone or in combination trial. J Clin Oncol. 2011;29(32):4266–72.

23. Sanoff HK, Goldberg RM. Colorectal cancer treatment in older patients. Gastrointest Cancer Res. 2007;1(6):248–53.

24. Faivre-Finn C, Benhamiche AM, Maingon P, et al. Changes in the practice of adjuvant radiotherapy in resectable rectal cancer within a French well-defined population. Radiother Oncol. 2000;57:137–42.
25. Ayanian JZ, Zaslavsky AM, Fuchs CS, et al. Use of adjuvant chemotherapy and radiation therapy for colorectal cancer in a population-based cohort. J Clin Oncol. 2003;21:1293–300.
26. Jung B, Påhlman L, Johansson R, Nilsson E. Rectal cancer treatment and outcome in the elderly: an audit based on the Swedish Rectal Cancer Registry 1995–2004. BMC Cancer. 2009;9:68.
27. Gagliardi G, Pucciarelli S, Asteria CR, et al. A nationwide audit of the use of radiotherapy for rectal cancer in Italy. Tech Coloproctol. 2010;14(3):229–35.
28. Aparicio T, Navazesh A, Boutron I, et al. Half of elderly patients routinely treated for colorectal cancer receive a sub-standard treatment. Crit Rev Oncol Hematol. 2009;71(3):249–57.
29. Quipourt V, Jooste V, Cottet V, Faivre J, Bouvier AM. Comorbidities alone do not explain the undertreatment of colorectal cancer in older adults: a French population-based study. J Am Geriatr Soc. 2011;59(4):694–8.
30. Holm T, Singnomklao T, Rutqvist LE, Cedermark B. Adjuvant preoperative radiotherapy in patients with rectal carcinoma. Adverse effects during long term follow-up of two randomized trials. Cancer. 1996;78(5):968–76.
31. Pignon T, Horiot JC, Bolla M, van Poppel H, Bartelink H, Roelofsen F, Pene F, Gerard A, Einhorn N, Nguyen TD, Vanglabbeke M, Scalliet P. Age is not a limiting factor for radical radiotherapy in pelvic malignancies. Radiother Oncol. 1997;42(2):107–20.
32. Kalata P, Martus P, Zettl H, Rödel C, Hohenberger W, Raab R, Becker H, Liersch T, Wittekind C, Sauer R, Fietkau R, German Rectal Cancer Study Group. Differences between clinical trial participants and patients in a population-based registry: the German Rectal Cancer Study vs. the Rostock Cancer Registry. Dis Colon Rectum. 2009;52(3):425–37.
33. Hutchins LF, Unger JM, Crowley JJ, et al. Underrepresentation of patients 65 years of age or older in cancer-treatment trials. N Engl J Med. 1999;341:2061–7.
34. Murthy VH, Krumholz HM, Gross CP. Participation in cancer clinical trials: race-, sex-, and age based disparities. JAMA. 2004;291:2720–6.
35. Sargent DJ, Goldberg RM, Jacobson SD, et al. A pooled analysis of adjuvant chemotherapy for resected colon cancer in elderly patients. N Engl J Med. 2001;345:1091–7.
36. Goldberg RM, Tabah-Fisch I, Bleiberg H, et al. Pooled analysis of safety and efficacy of oxaliplatin plus fluorouracil/leucovorin administered bimonthly in elderly patients with colorectal cancer. J Clin Oncol. 2006;24:4085–91.
37. Bujko K, Nowacki MP, Nasierowska-Guttmejer A, et al. Sphincter preservation following preoperative radiotherapy for rectal cancer: report of a randomized trial comparing short-term radiotherapy vs. conventionally fractionated radiochemotherapy. Radiother Oncol. 2004;72:15–24.
38. Swedish Rectal Cancer Trial: Initial report from a Swedish multicentre study examining the role of preoperative irradiation in the treatment of patients with resectable rectal carcinoma. Br J Surg. 1993; 80: 1333–6.
39. Ngan S, Fisher R, Goldstein D, et al. TROG, AGITG, CSSANZ, and RACS. A randomized trial comparing local recurrence (LR) rates between short-course (SC) and long-course (LC) preoperative radiotherapy (RT) for clinical T3 rectal cancer: an intergroup trial (TROG, AGITG, CSSANZ, RACS). J Clin Oncol. 2010;28(15 Suppl):abstract 3509.
40. Petersson D, Cedermark B, Holm T, Radu C, Påhlman L, Glimelius B, Martling A. Interim analysis of the Stockholm III trial of preoperative radiotherapy regimens for rectal cancer. Br J Surg. 2010;97(4):580–7.
41. Radu C, Berglund A, Pahlman L, Glimelius B. Short-course preoperative radiotherapy with delayed surgery in rectal cancer – a retrospective study. Radiother Oncol. 2008;87(3):343–9.
42. Hatfield P, Hingorani M, Radhakrishna G, Cooper R, Melcher A, Crellin A, Kwok-Williams M, Sebag-Montefiore D. Short-course radiotherapy, with elective delay prior to surgery, in patients with unresectable rectal cancer who have poor performance status or significant comorbidity. Radiother Oncol. 2009;92(2):210–4.

43. Paszat LF, Brundage MD, Groome PA, Schulze K, Mackillop WJ. A population-based study of rectal cancer: permanent colostomy as an outcome. Int J Radiat Oncol Biol Phys. 1999;45(5):1185–91.

44. Schrag D, Gelfand SE, Bach PB, Guillem J, Minsky BD, Begg CB. Who gets adjuvant treatment for stage II and III rectal cancer? Insight from surveillance, epidemiology, and end results—Medicare. J Clin Oncol. 2001;19(17):3712–8.

45. Schroen AT, Cress RD. Use of surgical procedures and adjuvant therapy in rectal cancer treatment: a population-based study. Ann Surg. 2001;234(5):641–51.

46. Neugut AI, Fleischauer AT, Sundararajan V, et al. Use of adjuvant chemotherapy and radiation therapy for rectal canceramong the elderly: a population-based study. J Clin Oncol. 2002;20:2643–50.

47. Dharma-Wardene MW, de Gara C, Au HJ, Hanson J, Hatcher J. Ageism in rectal carcinoma? Treatment and outcome variations. Int J Gastrointest Cancer. 2002;32(2–3):129–38.

48. Phelip JM, Milan C, Herbert C, Grosclaude P, Arveux P, Raverdy N, Daures JP, Faivre J. Evaluation of the management of rectal cancers before and after the consensus conference in France. Eur J Gastroenterol Hepatol. 2004;16(10):1003–9.

49. Baxter NN, Rothenberger DA, Morris AM, Bullard KM. Adjuvant radiation for rectal cancer: do we measure up to the standard of care? An epidemiologic analysis of trends over 25 years in the United States. Dis Colon Rectum. 2005;48(1):9–15.

50. Vulto AJ, Lemmens VE, Louwman MW, et al. The influence of age and co-morbidity on receiving radiotherapy as part of primary treatment for cancer in south Netherlands, 1995–2002. Cancer. 2006;106:2734–42.

51. Larsen SG, Wiig JN, Tretli S, Giercksky KE. Surgery and pre-operative irradiation for locally advanced or recurrent rectal cancer in patients over 75 years of age. Colorectal Dis. 2006;8(3):177–85.

52. Wolff HA, Conradi LC, Schirmer M, Beissbarth T, Sprenger T, Rave-Fränk M, Hennies S, Hess CF, Becker H, Christiansen H, Liersch T. Gender-specific acute organ toxicity during intensified preoperative radiochemotherapy for rectal cancer. Oncologist. 2011;16(5):621–31.

53. Lorchel F, Peignaux K, Créhange G, Bosset M, Puyraveau M, Mercier M, Bosset JF, Maingon P. Preoperative radiotherapy in elderly patients with rectal cancer. Gastroenterol Clin Biol. 2007;31(4):436–41.

54. Pasetto LM, Basso U, Friso ML, et al. Determining therapeutic approaches in the elderly with rectal cancer. Drugs Aging. 2007;24(9):781–90.

55. Fiorica F, Cartei F, Carau B, Berretta S, Spartà D, Tirelli U, Santangelo A, Maugeri D, Luca S, Leotta C, Sorace R, Berretta M. Adjuvant radiotherapy on older and oldest elderly rectal cancer patients. Arch Gerontol Geriatr. 2009;49(1):54–9.

56. Margalit DN, Mamom HJ, Ancukiewicz M, et al. Tolerability of combined modality therapy for rectal cancer in elderly patients aged 75 years and older. Int J Radiat Oncol Biol Phys. 2011;81(5):e735–41.

57. Seymour MT, Thompson LC, Wasan HS, Middleton G, Brewster AE, Shepherd SF, O'Mahony MS, Maughan TS, Parmar M, Langley RE, FOCUS2 Investigators; National Cancer Research Institute Colorectal Cancer Clinical Studies Group. Chemotherapy options in elderly and frail patients with metastatic colorectal cancer (MRC FOCUS2): an open-label, randomized factorial trial. Lancet. 2011;377(9779):1749–59.

58. Peeters KC, van de Velde CJ, Leer JW, Martijn H, Junggeburt JM, Kranenbarg EK, Steup WH, Wiggers T, Rutten HJ, Marijnen CA. Late side effects of short-course preoperative radiotherapy combined with total mesorectal excision for rectal cancer: increased bowel dysfunction in irradiated patients–a Dutch colorectal cancer group study. J Clin Oncol. 2005;23(25):6199–206.

59. Bacon C, Giovannucci E, Testa M, et al. The association of treatment-related symptoms with quality-of-life outcomes for localized prostate carcinoma patients. Cancer. 2002;94:862–71.

60. Andreyev HJ. Gastrointestinal problems following pelvic radiotherapy: the past, the present and the future. Clin Oncol (R Coll Radiol). 2007;19:790–9.

61. Pucciarelli S, Gagliardi G, Maretto I, et al. Long-term oncologic results and complications after preoperative chemoradiotherapy for rectal cancer: a single-institution experience after a median follow-up of 95 months. Ann Surg Oncol. 2009;16(4):893–9.
62. Lange MM, van de Velde CJ. Faecal and urinary incontinence after multimodality treatment of rectal cancer. PLoS Med. 2008;5(10):e202.
63. Lönn S, Gilbert ES, Ron E, et al. Comparison of second cancer risks from brachytherapy and external beam therapy after uterine corpus cancer. Cancer Epidemiol Biomarkers Prev. 2010;19(2):464–74.
64. Bouvier AM, Jooste V, Bonnetain F, et al. Adjuvant treatments do not alter the quality of life in elderly patients with colorectal cancer: a population-based study. Cancer. 2008;113(4): 879–86.
65. Boige V, Mendiboure J, Pignon JP, et al. Pharmacogenetic assessment of toxicity and outcome in patients with metastatic colorectal cancer treated with LV5FU2, FOLFOX, and FOLFIRI: FFCD 2000–05. J Clin Oncol. 2010;28:2556–64.
66. Agostini M, Pasetto LM, Pucciarelli S, Terrazzino S, Ambrosi A, Bedin C, Galdi F, Friso ML, Mescoli C, Urso E, Leon A, Lise M, Nitti D. Glutathione S-transferase P1 Ile105Val polymorphism is associated with haematological toxicity in elderly rectal cancer patients receiving preoperative chemoradiotherapy. Drugs Aging. 2008;25(6):531–9.
67. Vuong T, Belliveau PJ, Michel RP, Moftah BA, Parent J, Trudel JL, Reinhold C, Souhami L. Conformal preoperative endorectal brachytherapy treatment for locally advanced rectal cancer: early results of a phase I/II study. Dis Colon Rectum. 2002;45:1486–93.
68. Kaufman N, Nori D, Shank B, Linares L, Harrison L, Fass D, Enker W. Remote afterloading intraluminal brachytherapy in the treatment of rectal, rectosigmoid, and anal cancer: a feasibility study. Int J Radiat Oncol Biol Phys. 1989;17:663–8.
69. Jakobsen A, Mortensen JP, Bisgaard C, Lindebjerg J, Hansen JW, Rafaelsen SR. Preoperative chemoradiation of locally advanced T3 rectal cancer combined with an endorectal boost. Int J Radiat Oncol Biol Phys. 2006;64:461–5.
70. Corner C, Bryant L, Chapman C, Glynne-Jones R, Hoskin PJ. High-dose-rate afterloading intraluminal brachytherapy for advanced inoperable rectal carcinoma. Brachytherapy. 2010;9:66–70.
71. Tunio MA, Rafi M, Hashmi A, et al. High-dose-rate intraluminal brachytherapy during preoperative chemoradiation for locally advanced rectal cancers. World J Gastroenterol. 2010;16(35): 4436–42.
72. Cesari M, et al. Fraility syndrome and skeletal muscle: results from the Invecchiare in Chianti study. Am J Clin Nutr. 2006;83:1142–8.
73. Charlson M, et al. A new method of classifying prognostic comorbidity in longitudinal studies: development and validation. J Chronic Dis. 1987;40:373–83.
74. Extermann M, Hurria A. Comprehensive geriatric assessment for older patients with cancer. J Clin Oncol. 2007;25:1824–31.
75. Extermann M, Overcash J, Lyman G, et al. Comorbidity and functional status are independent in older cancer patients. J Clin Oncol. 1998;16:1582–7.
76. Chen H, Overcash J, Extermann M, et al. Comprehensive geriatric assessment in elderly cancer patients: impact on overall survival and progression free survival. Poster P76. In: American Geriatric Society meeting, Philadelphia, 19–23 May 1999.
77. Saliba D, et al. The vulnerable elders survey: a tool for identifying vulnerable older people in the community. J Am Geriatr Soc. 2001;49:1691–9.
78. Rodin MB, Mohile SG. A practical approach to geriatric assessment in oncology. J Clin Oncol. 2007;25:1936–44.
79. Mohile SG, et al. A pilot study of the vulnerable elders survey-13 compared with the comprehensive geriatric assessment for identifying disability in older patients with prostate cancer who receive androgen ablation. Cancer. 2007;109:802–10.

Chapter 10
Adjuvant Therapy of Colorectal Cancer in Older People

Aimery de Gramont, Leila Bengrine-Lefevre, May Mabro, and Elisabeth Carola

Abstract Colorectal cancer (CRC) is the fourth cause of cancer deaths. More than one-third of colon cancers are stage III at presentation; their 5-year relative survival is 69 %.

Among the high-incidence cancers, CRC has the highest median age at presentation. Thus, the administration of adjuvant therapy after curative surgery for elderly patients remains a burning question in daily practice.

In the adjuvant setting, while there is an advantage in relapse-free survival with adjuvant therapy, there is no evidence-based survival benefit for adjuvant therapy due to confounding non-cancer-related deaths. However, with an optimal and careful management of relapses or second cancers, a survival benefit with adjuvant therapy is possible in some elderly patients. The use of a comprehensive geriatric assessment is strongly recommended to evaluate chemotherapy appropriateness. Elderly patients with good physical condition are able to receive combination therapy in a similar fashion to younger patients.

Keywords Colorectal cancer • Elderly • Stage III • Adjuvant chemotherapy • Fluoropyrimidines • Oxaliplatin • Older patients • Recurrence • Survival

A. de Gramont, M.D. (✉)
Department of Medical Oncology, GERCOR, Paris, France

Department of Medical Oncology, Hopital Saint-Antoine,
184 rue du Faubourg Saint Antoine, Paris 75012, France
e-mail: aimery.de-gramont@sat.aphp.fr

L. Bengrine-Lefevre, M.D.
Oncology Department, Saint Antoine Hospital, Paris 75012, France

M. Mabro, M.D.
Oncologie, Hopital Foch, Suresnes 92150, France

E. Carola, M.D.
Oncologie Médicale, GHPSO, Senlis 60300, France

D. Papamichael, R.A. Audisio (eds.), *Management of Colorectal Cancers in Older People*, 111
DOI 10.1007/978-0-85729-984-0_10, © Springer-Verlag London 2013

Introduction

The estimated worldwide incidence of colorectal cancer (CRC) reached 1.23 million in 2008. Colorectal cancer is the third among all cancers in incidence, just after lung and breast cancers [1]. It also represents the fourth cause of cancer deaths after lung, gastric, and liver cancers. Colorectal cancers are more frequent in developed countries. While increasing in some countries, especially in Asia, CRC incidence is decreasing in the USA, from 66.3 cases per 100,000 persons in 1985 to 45.3 in 2007 [2]. This decline is attributed to CRC screening and removal of colorectal polyps before they progress to cancer.

Approximately 70–80 % of the CRC cases are colon or high rectal cancer, defined by the presence of the inferior pole of the tumor above the peritoneal reflection that is at least 15 cm from the anal margin or by a distal end of the tumor more than 12 cm from the anal verge [3, 4]. Low or medium rectum accounts for 20–30 % of the CRC cases.

CRC cancers are classified at presentation in five stages [5]. Briefly, stage 0 is carcinoma in situ, involving only the mucosa; stage I is a cancer extended through the muscularis mucosa into the submucosa or into the muscularis propria; stage II is a cancer grown into the outermost layers of the colon or through the wall of the colon or rectum but has not spread to lymph nodes; stage III is a cancer that has spread to lymph nodes but has no metastases; stage IV or advanced colorectal cancer is a metastatic cancer. The full American Joint Committee in Cancer (AJCC) classification, which has been recently updated, further subclassifies stages II and III [5].

At diagnosis, in the USA, excluding stage 0, stage I and II account for 39 % of all CRC cases; stage III, 37 %; stage IV, 20 %; and the remaining 5 % were unstaged. Their 5-year relative survivals (deaths of colorectal cancer only) were 90, 69, 12, and 33 %, respectively [6]. Following the decline in incidence, colorectal cancer death rate is slowly declining since 1950 in females and since 1985 in males. The decline accelerated from 1998 to 2007 and is estimated at 2.9 % per year in men and 2.2 % per year in women.

Based on these data, the medical management of CRC cancer differs according to the stage. Obviously, adjuvant therapy to prevent recurrence has no place in stage I and in many of the stage II considered as low risk. However, adjuvant therapy is an important part of the CRC management in high-risk stage II and in stage III.

The particularity of CRC is a median age at diagnosis of 71 years and more than 25 % of the cases are diagnosed at age over 75 years [2]. Among the previously cited high-incidence cancers, CRC has the highest median age at presentation. Thus, the administration of adjuvant therapy after curative surgery or palliative therapy for elderly patients with CRC remains as a burning question in daily practice.

The Geriatric Assessment

Like in other cancers, the elderly population with colon cancer is not homogeneous regarding physiologic age, comorbidities, and living conditions. Ideally, the geriatric assessment in adjuvant colon cancer should follow three steps:

The first is a general evaluation of the life expectancy. A nonspecific evaluation, such as the Lee's prognostic index is appropriate [7].

The goal of the second step is to identify the patients who will benefit from a comprehensive geriatric assessment (CGA). CGA is time consuming and sometimes not available in a time frame consistent with the management of newly diagnosed cancer. A pilot study evaluated the interest of achieving a mini-geriatric assessment by the gastroenterologist prior to therapeutic decision. Treatment was adapted to 47 % of cancer cases in view of the results of this mini-geriatric assessment. When no change in oncologic care was required, a change in the non-oncologic care has been proposed in 72 % of patients and social measures in 38 % of cases [8]. Several teams are currently working on the validation of tools for "screening" to identify patients who require a CGA. In France, the objective of the "Oncodage" trial is to validate a questionnaire entitled "G8" to, quickly and safely, detect if a CGA is necessary to establish a treatment [9]. G8 takes seven items of the MNA (mini nutritional assessment) plus chronological age. Other approaches are under experimentation, such as the aCGA score (abbreviated comprehensive geriatric assessment) developed in the USA (Tampa, Florida) [10] or by using other concepts than CGA including the five criteria of frailty phenotype described by Fried (weakness, poor endurance, reduced physical activity, slow walking speed, and unintentional weight loss over the past year) [11, 12]. Some of these tools should be validated in the coming years.

The third step is the CGA. CGA can improve the prognosis of elderly patients with cancer particularly among patients with advanced cancer [13]. Some areas of the CGA seem predictive of morbidity and mortality: a recent study showed that malnutrition was the main poor prognostic factor for survival of elderly patients with cancer [14]. In breast cancer, it was demonstrated by two prospective studies that CGA altered the oncology care in nearly 40 % of cases [15, 16]. In CRC, in addition to CGA, some diseases will have to be specifically evaluated according to the proposed chemotherapy. For example, the systematic searches for a preexisting neuropathy in case of chemotherapy with oxaliplatin, for hypoalbuminemia in case of treatment with irinotecan, for an abnormal renal function in case of treatment with capecitabine, as well as a careful examination of the skin before EGFR-targeted therapy, are essential to anticipate some specific potential toxicities.

Then, patients who should have cancer therapeutic adaptation have to be identified. This identification is still empirical. A decision tree classifying patients into three groups for which the therapeutic approach is different has been proposed by Balducci [17]. Patients called "harmonious" with no comorbidity or dependence are candidates for active treatment of their disease. A priori, this active treatment can be the standard treatment, the same that would be offered to younger patients. Fragile patients (defined by a decrease of at least one activity of daily life in ADL score, the presence of at least three comorbidities, at least one geriatric syndrome such as trouble walking or falling, incontinence, mental confusion or dementia, denutrition) are not able to receive an active treatment of their tumors and must be symptomatically treated. In patients identified "intermediary" with the presence of one or two comorbidities or dependence in instrumental activities of daily living (IADL score), the therapeutic decision depends on the life expectancy of the patient: specific tumor therapy is indicated if life expectancy is linked to cancer and predictable tolerance of chemotherapy is good. These criteria must be modulated according to the intensity of care which varies with the stage. These criteria are indicative because currently there is no study showing their contribution in the management of colorectal cancers. Data coming from a FFCD study in metastatic colorectal cancer and the GERCOR OLD-07 study, with a significant contingent of adjuvant colorectal cancer patients, may help to define the predictive factors of safety and efficacy of chemotherapy in this setting.

Based on the geriatricians' definition of frailty, the elderly CRC population is divided in three groups: fit (or harmonious), non-fit but non-frail (or intermediary, vulnerable), and frail (or fragile) patients [18]. The geriatric assessment based on general scales can quite easily recognize both the fit population who can receive the same treatment as the younger patients and the frail population with age-related comorbidities, such as impaired renal, cardiac, and liver function; general decline in health; and loss of autonomy and cognitive impairment, who should not receive chemotherapy. However, the problem is the optimal management of the non-fit but non-frail population. Thus, a specific tool based on the geriatric assessment but also adapted to the acceptance and tolerance of the various chemotherapy regimens used in CRC is needed to optimally manage the elderly patients. New scales like the CRASH score (Chemotherapy Risk Assessment Scale for High-Age Patients) have been proposed, based on observed toxicities with different chemotherapy regimens and the patient risk [19]. Other efforts are being done in prospective studies such as the ongoing GERCOR OLD 1 trial. The new scale in experimentation combines general condition and CRC clinical and biological items with a simplified ten-item geriatric questionnaire. The goal is to validate the predictive value of this new scale in terms of safety and efficacy of the administered chemotherapy regimen. Furthermore, if the fit population can receive the same regimens as the younger patients, the same therapeutic strategy may not be applicable. The ability to receive several therapy lines in case of relapse may differ between the fit older patients and the younger patients.

All these considerations can all impact the therapeutic decision, especially when the patient's family and physician are involved [20]. Of note, the main reasons for not including patients in a clinical trial are physician- and not patient-related [20–22]. When asked if they were willing to accept chemotherapy, between 88 and 100 % of elderly (>70 years) cancer patients would accept a mild chemotherapy and even 70–78 % would accept a strong chemotherapy [23].

Adjuvant Therapy

Women and men who reach 70 years have an additional median life expectancy of approximately 15 and 10 years, respectively [24]. The risk of relapse is maximal during the three 1st years after surgery and the peak is at 18 months [25]. This

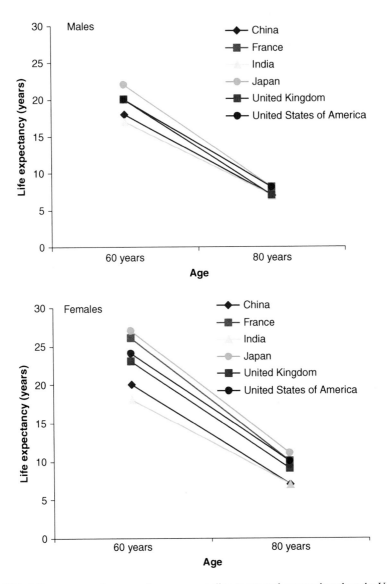

Fig. 10.1 Life expectancy in men and women according to age and country based on the United Nations data [24]

difference between time to relapse and life expectancy suggests that adjuvant chemotherapy should be considered for the majority of elderly patients, especially in women who have the longest life expectancy after 70 years. Figure 10.1 illustrates the life expectancy in men and women according to age and country based on the United Nations data [24].

Experience of Adjuvant Therapy in the Elderly Patients

Unfortunately, elderly patients are underrepresented in the randomized studies [20]. For example, in the recent adjuvant phase III, only 14–24 % of the population was >70 years and very few over 75 years. This proportion remains stable with time (Table 10.1). Furthermore, all these patients had per protocol a good performance status and limited comorbidities to be included in the trials (Table 10.2) [3].

In trials, adjuvant therapy has shown a strong benefit in stage III patients and is still controversial in stage II patients [3, 4, 30–32]. Fluoropyrimidines alone, either leucovorin/5-FU or capecitabine, have improved survival in patients with stage III colon cancer with mild toxicity when 5-FU is used as infusion or with oral capecitabine [29, 33–35]. However, the most active regimens for stage III patients are FOLFOX or XELOX, having shown superiority over fluoropyrimidines in three large studies [3, 4, 30, 31]. In stage II patients, fluoropyrimidines are the standard therapy in patients without deficient mismatch repair (dMMR) [36]. FOLFOX might be considered in high-risk stage II, especially those who have T4b tumors (tumor has grown through the wall of the colon or rectum and is attached to or invades into nearby tissues or organs) [30]. Of note, patients with dMMR do better without chemotherapy [37]. Like irinotecan, targeted therapies in the adjuvant setting, either bevacizumab or cetuximab, failed in combination with chemotherapy [38–40].

Pooled analysis of adjuvant trials in colon cancer patients demonstrated that selected patients older than 70 years received the same benefit from adjuvant therapy based on 5-fluorouracil (5-FU) with leucovorin (LV) or levamisole as younger counterparts [41]. However, in this study, 13.4 % of the elderly patients (>70 years) died without recurrence vs. only 4.7 % of the younger patients, already showing the impact of other diseases in this population. A large population-based cohort study of 3,357 elderly patients (>67 years, median 74 years) according to the Surveillance, Epidemiology and End Results (SEER) registry also demonstrated the advantage of adjuvant chemotherapy with fluoropyrimidine-based chemotherapy in the stage III elderly patients: 5-FU reduced the hazard of death by 27 %, an absolute benefit of 12 % over matched untreated patients [42].

Table 10.1 Patients ≥70 years included in recent adjuvant trials according to the year of the first inclusion

Trial	Accrual period	# pts	% pts ≥70 years	Experimental treatment arm[a]	% stage III[b]
MOSAIC [3]	1998–2001	2,246	14	FOLFOX4	60
NSABP C-07 [4]	2000–2002	2,434	16	FLOX	71
CALGB 89803 [26]	1999–2001	1,263	24	IFL	98
PETACC-3 [27]	2000–2002	3,186	13	FOLFIRI	71
NSABP C-06 [28]	1997–1999	1,557	22	Uracil/tegafur	53
X-ACT [29]	1998–2001	1,983	20	Capecitabine	100

[a]Compared to control arm of intravenous 5-flourouracil (IV 5-FU) and leucovorin (LV)
[b]Remaining patients were stage II or unknown

Table 10.2 Example of non-cancer-related inclusion and exclusion criteria in a randomized study

---

Inclusion criteria

Histologically proven stage Dukes « B2 » (stage II: T3–T4 N0 M0) and « C » (stage III: any T N1–2 M0) colon carcinoma. The inferior pole of the tumor must be above the peritoneal reflection (>15 cm from the anal margin)

Patients must have undergone complete resection of the primary tumor without gross or microscopic evidence of residual disease

Patients must be randomized in the study in order to start treatment within 7 weeks after surgery

Age 18–75 years old

PS < 2 (Karnofsky ≥60 %)

No previous chemotherapy, immunotherapy, or radiotherapy

No biological major abnormalities : absolute neutrophil count >1.5 × 10^9/l, platelets >100 × 109/l, serum creatinine <1.25 times the upper limit of normal, total bilirubin, ASAT / ALAT <2 times the upper limit of the normal range, CEA <10 ng/ml

Documentation of a negative pregnancy test must be available for premenopausal women with intact reproductive organs

Men and women who are fertile must use a medically acceptable contraceptive throughout the treatment period and for 3 months following cessation of treatment with oxaliplatin

Subjects must be made aware, before entering this trial, of the risk of becoming pregnant or in fathering children

Signed informed consent obtained prior to study entry

Exclusion criteria

Pregnant or lactating women

Women of child-bearing potential not using a contraceptive method

Previous cancer of the colon or rectum

Previous malignancies other than adequately treated in situ carcinoma of the uterine cervix or basal or squamous cell carcinoma of the skin, unless there has been a disease-free interval of at least 10 years

Participation in another clinical trial with any investigational drug within 30 days prior to randomization

Peripheral neuropathy (NCI CTC ≥grade I)

Uncontrolled congestive heart failure or angina pectoris, or hypertension or arrhythmia

History of significant neurologic or psychiatric disorders

Active infection

MOSAIC [3]

PS performance status

Of note, in observational studies or daily practice, the use of adjuvant chemotherapy in elderly patients is somewhat different to that investigated in the trials. Among patients included in another observational study of adjuvant chemotherapy in the USA, only 50 % of the patients over 75 years with stage III colon cancer received adjuvant chemotherapy. They received less toxic and shorter chemotherapy regimens compared with younger counterparts [43]. Interestingly, the elderly patients had fewer adverse events than younger patients. Selection of less vulnerable patients may have contributed to the fact that older patients tolerate adjuvant chemotherapy better than younger patients.

Table 10.3 Hazard ratios for disease-free survival (DFS) and overall survival (OS) in the elderly subpopulation in recent studies

	$N>70$	%	DFS HR	OS HR	Reference
ACCENT Oral FP	755	21.3	1.13	1.17	[44]
X-ACT	397[a]	20.0	0.93[b]	0.93[b]	[29]
C-06	358	22.3	NA>(1.13)	NA>(1.17)	[28]
ACCENT Oxaliplatin	703	15.0	1.04	1.19	
MOSAIC	315[c]	14.0	0.91	1.10	[45]
C-07	388	16.9	NA>(1.04)	NA>(1.19)	[4]
XELOXA	409[a]	21.7	0.87	0.94	[46]

[a]Stage III only
[b]Estimated from forest plot
[c]Stage III 190 patients

In elderly patients, the addition of oxaliplatin to fluoropyrimidine-based chemotherapy constitutes an important question in the daily therapeutic decision process. In a pooled analysis of NSABP-C07 and MOSAIC trials for stage II and III, oxaliplatin-based chemotherapy was not superior to FU/LV in patients ≥70 years for disease-free survival (DFS) or overall survival (OS) [44]. These data challenged the benefit of oxaliplatin in this subcategory of patients (Table 10.3). However, these trials are different: Interaction between age and therapy for OS was significant in NSABP-C07, but not in MOSAIC [47]. This might be due to the toxicity of the FLOX regimen used in NSABP-C07. This regimen which combines 5-FU as a bolus with oxaliplatin had a high incidence of grade 3–4 diarrhea (36.9 %) and dehydration (11.3 %) that was not observed in MOSAIC. Patients older than 60 years were also at risk for bowel wall injury (6.7 %) after treatment with FLOX [4]. The results of the NO16968 trial (XELOXA) in the elderly population, comparing 5-FU/LV and XELOX, have shown comparable results in young and elderly populations [46, 48].

In the MOSAIC trial, we found that fewer patients between 70 and 75 years had surgery for metastases and fewer had irinotecan or oxaliplatin-based therapy at relapse in the FOLFOX4 arm than in the LV5FU2 arm of the trial. More deaths not related to colon cancer also occurred with FOLFOX4, including a significant number of second cancer deaths [45]. The finding of a lower management of late events after combination chemotherapy in elderly patients may explain the DFS and OS benefit with FOLFOX4 of less magnitude than in younger patients. If it is patient- or physician-related remains to be demonstrated. We also observed an unexpected difference according to sex, females doing better on oxaliplatin than males, with all the restriction of a retrospective analysis on a small population (Fig. 10.2). Greater life expectancy and better general condition of women 70–75 years than men at the same age can explain this finding. This suggests considering the gender in the adjuvant management of elderly patients with colon cancer.

Finally, in our opinion, adjuvant therapy with FOLFOX/XELOX in the fit elderly patients remains an option in a selected population, with a careful management of comorbidities, side effects, relapse, and second cancers. A reduced

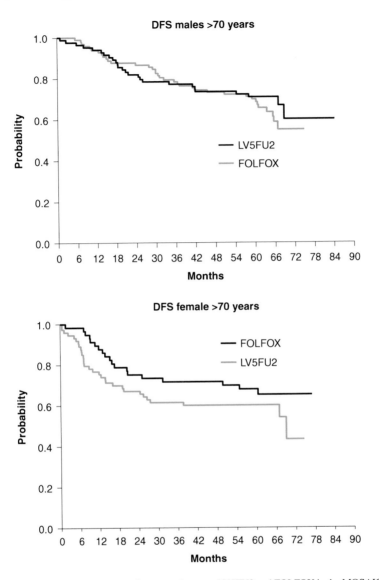

Fig. 10.2 Disease-free survival according to sex between LV5FU2 and FOLFOX in the MOSAIC trial

duration of adjuvant chemotherapy has been suggested to improve tolerability in elderly patients. In this regard, the IDEA project (International Duration Evaluation of Adjuvant Chemotherapy) is comparing 3–6 months of FOLFOX or XELOX in more than 10,000 stage III patients in different clinical trials evaluating this concept. The analysis of the elderly population included in this project will provide strong input to determine whether a short adjuvant treatment may be of benefit. Figure 10.3 represents the adjuvant chemotherapy regimens discussed in this chapter.

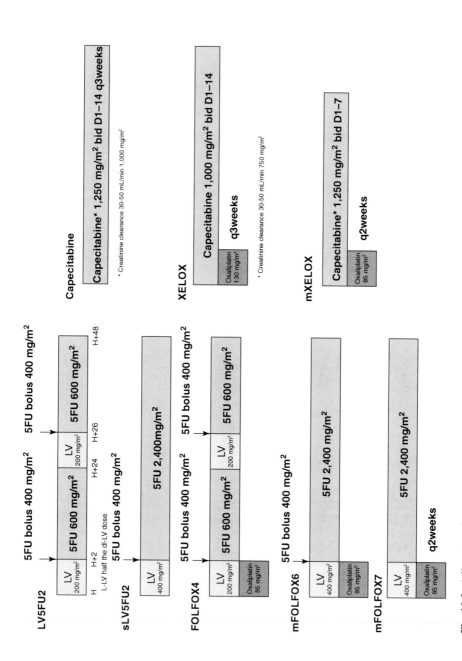

Fig. 10.3 Adjuvant regimens

Table 10.4 Evaluation process and management of elderly patient with adjuvant colon cancer

Lee's prognostic index 4-year life expectancy (%)	Patient's condition	Management
<50	Frail or vulnerable	No adjuvant therapy
>50	Vulnerable or fit	Adjuvant therapy can be considered
50–80	Vulnerable	CGA: no adjuvant therapy or, if mandatory, crash test and adapted adjuvant regimen
	Further testing gives poor results: G8 < 14 and/or VES13 > 3	
	Further testing gives good results: G8 > 14 et/ou VES13 < 3	Crash test: adapted adjuvant regimen
>80	Patient is fit	Standard adjuvant regimen

Practical Management of Colon Cancer in the Elderly Patients

The practical management of these patients is based on the evaluations of the general condition of the patient, of the cancer risk, and of the potential toxicity of the regimen (Table 10.4).

Evaluating the General Condition of the Elderly Patient

The first step is to estimate the life expectancy in all patients over 70 years of age. The Lee's prognostic index can be used first. Further onco-geriatric evaluation is mandatory for all patients that are either non-frail or non-fit; it can be G8 test or the Vulnerable Elders Survey (VES-13) then CGA [7, 9, 15, 49, 50]. CGA is also recommended in the very old patients and in case of limited experience in geriatric oncology. The comprehensive geriatric assessment can recognize potentially treatable conditions that may lessen the tolerance of cancer treatment and be reversed with proper intervention [17].

The goal is to identify to which group belongs a patient:

- Fit: patient with no comorbidity, good health performance status, no physical dependence, and no cognitive impairment.
- Vulnerable: patient with some comorbidities and few dependences. It is very important to assess the reversible geriatric problems before deciding the oncologic treatment.
- Frail: patient with important geriatric syndrome. In this condition, the palliative treatment is best supportive care.

Table 10.5 Potential survival results according to stage and therapy in 2012

Stage	Prognostic markers	Full therapy 3-year DFS (%)	Low toxicity therapy 3-year DFS (%)	No chemotherapy 3-year DFS (%)
II low risk	dMMR	90	90	87
II high risk	T4b	85	80	75
III	N invaded lymph nodes	78	73	60

Based on MOSAIC data [3], FOLFOX, and 5-FU arms for stages II and III
dMMR deficient mismatch repair

Evaluating the Potential of Chemotherapy

This evaluation is based on the prognosis of cancer and the potential therapeutic benefit. As previously discussed, this knowledge is based on the experience in trials that have included a limited number of elderly patients. Of note, stage II patients with dMMR may have a detrimental effect of adjuvant chemotherapy with fluoropyrimidines alone [37]. Table 10.5 summarizes the potential of therapy according to stage and therapy.

Evaluating the Safety Profile of the Regimen

Another goal is to evaluate the risk of chemotherapy toxicity. Table 10.6 summarizes grade 3/4 toxicities observed in the adjuvant trials in elderly patients. These results concerned only the fit elderly patients. LV5FU2 is the safer regimen with little severe toxicity and none occurring in more than 10 % of the patients. Oral capecitabine is the most convenient, but may not be suitable in elderly patients with some cognitive impairment and has diarrhea and hand-foot syndrome as limiting toxicities occurring in 13 and 20 % of the patients, respectively. Oral capecitabine recommended dose in elderly patients is 1,250 mg/m^2 twice daily on days 1–14, every 3 weeks. Patients with a creatinine clearance of 30–50 mL/min should receive a dose of 950 mg/m^2 twice daily [53]. FOLFOX and XELOX have more toxicities than fluoropyrimidines alone, limiting toxicities being neurosensory for both, neutropenia for FOLFOX4, and diarrhea for XELOX. In fit or vulnerable elderly patients, modified FOLFOX6 with a single bolus 5-FU or a modified FOLFOX7 without bolus 5-FU and oxaliplatin 85 mg/m^2 can further reduce the toxicity. Modified XELOX with capecabine 1 week on, 1 week off and oxaliplatin 85 mg/m^2 every 2 weeks could also be more suitable in elderly patients than the recommended 3-weekly XELOX [54] (Fig. 10.3).

New scales like the CRASH score (Chemotherapy Risk Assessment Scale for High-Age Patients) have been proposed, based on observed toxicities with different chemotherapy regimens and the patient risk [19]. As previously exposed, GERCOR is developing another simplified scale, specific to colon cancer. In addition, all the supportive measures to help tolerating chemotherapy should be offered [17].

Table 10.6 Safety of adjuvant chemotherapy in elderly patients (grade 3/4 toxicities)

	LV5FU2	Capecitabine	FOLFOX	XELOX
Study	MOSAIC[a]	X-ACT [29]	MOSAIC [3, 30]	XELOXA [46, 52]
Population	151	397	155	190
Age (years)	70–76	>65	70–76	70–83
Stage	II–III	III	II–III	III
Neutropenia (%)	4	3	48	10
Febrile neutropenia (%)	0.7	0.3	2	<1
Thrombocytopenia (%)	0.7	1.8	1	5
Diarrhea (%)	9	13	12	26
Nausea/vomiting (%)	0.7	1	5	8
Mucositis (%)	2	3	1[a]	1
Hand-foot syndrome (%)	1.3	20	1[a]	4
Neurosensory (%)	0	0	12	11
All grade 3/4 (%)	13	NR	66	70
Grade 5 (%)	0.6	0.3	0.6[a]	0.6

NR not reported

[a]Unpublished data, courtesy of GERCOR

Guidelines for Adjuvant Colon Cancer Therapy

The goal of adjuvant therapy is to cure as many patients as possible. The normal duration of chemotherapy is 6 months.

The fit patients can tolerate the same regimen as the younger patients. However, as previously discussed, the benefit of FOLFOX/XELOX chemotherapy in OS and even DFS is less than in younger patients, the elderly facing deaths from other causes and often being unable to receive the optimal treatment in case of relapse or second cancer. As the benefit of chemotherapy is maintained in relapse-free survival (deaths of other causes than colon cancer are excluded in the definition, unlike DFS), the challenge is to identify the patients that may benefit from adjuvant therapy. For these reasons, it might be reasonable to select high- or intermediate-risk stage III and PS 0 patients (stage ≥T4N1b or ≥T3N2a), especially women for oxaliplatin/fluoropyrimidine therapy [55]. The two other options are either 3 months of oxaliplatin/fluoropyrimidines followed by 3 months of fluoropyrimidines or fluoropyrimidines alone. Adjuvant therapy can be recommended to only a fraction of stage II patients, like T4b with proficient MMR tumor, these patients having a worse prognostic than some stage III.

The non-fit non-frail patients with a life expectancy over 50 % at 4 years can receive fluoropyrimidines alone in case of stage III or high-risk stage II.

Treatment of low or medium rectum that can require preoperative radiotherapy should probably follow the same approach as colon cancer, even if the benefit of systemic chemotherapy is not formally established in this setting.

In a near future, prognostic and predictive biomarkers, including gene signature, will help us to better select the adjuvant treatment in elderly like in the younger patients [56–58].

Conclusion

There is a great heterogeneity within the elderly population in regard to overall health status, comorbidities, and performance status. The use of a comprehensive geriatric assessment is strongly recommended to evaluate chemotherapy appropriateness. Elderly patients with good physical condition are able to receive combination therapy in a similar fashion to younger patients. Careful monitoring for toxicity and rapid intervention when toxicity occurs is a mandatory component of optimal care, particularly in older patients. In the adjuvant setting, optimal and careful management of relapses or second cancers is required to observe the survival benefit in the elderly patients, as it is in the global population with colon cancer. With respect to clinical practice, age itself should not exclude treatment in elderly patients.

References

1. UN Data. http://globocan.iarc.fr/summary_table_pop.asp. Accessed on December 4, 2012
2. American Cancer Society. Cancer facts and figures 2012. http://seehttp://www.cancer.org/acs/groups/content/@epidemiologysurveilance/documents/document/acspc-029771.pdf. http://www.cancer.org/acs/groups/content/@epidemiologysurveilance/documents/document/acspc-031941.pdf. Accessed on December 4, 2012.
3. André T, Boni C, Mounedji-Boudiaf L, et al. Oxaliplatin, fluorouracil, and leucovorin as adjuvant treatment for colon cancer. N Engl J Med. 2004;350:2343–51.
4. Kuebler JP, Wieand HS, O'Connell MJ, et al. Oxaliplatin combined with weekly bolus fluorouracil and leucovorin as surgical adjuvant chemotherapy for stage II and III colon cancer: results from NSABP C-07. J Clin Oncol. 2007;25:2198–204.
5. American Joint Committee on Cancer. AJCC cancer staging manual. 7th ed. New York: Springer; 2010.
6. Chou JF, Row D, Gonen M, et al. Clinical and pathologic factors that predict lymph node yield from surgical specimens in colorectal cancer: a population-based study. Cancer. 2010;116:2560–70.
7. Lee SJ, Lindquist K, Segal MR, et al. Development and validation of a prognostic index for 4-year mortality in older adults. JAMA. 2006;295:801–8.
8. Aparicio T, Girard L, Bouarioua N, et al. A mini geriatric assessment helps treatment decision in elderly patients with digestive cancer. A pilot study. Crit Rev Oncol Hematol. 2011;77:63–9.
9. Artaud F, Bellera C, Rainfray M, et al. Performance evaluation of screening tools in oncogeriatrics in a national ONCODAGE multicenter study from the national. Bull Cancer. 2011;98:S69–70.
10. Overcash JA, Beckstead J, Extermann M, et al. The abbreviated comprehensive geriatric assessment (aCGA): a retrospective analysis. Crit Rev Oncol Hematol. 2005;54:129–36.
11. Fried LP, Tangen CM, Walston J, et al. Frailty in older adults: evidence for a phenotype. J Gerontol A Biol Sci Med Sci. 2001;56:M146–56.
12. Retornaz F, Monette J, Batist G, et al. Usefulness of frailty markers in the assessment of the health and functional status of older cancer patients referred for chemotherapy: a pilot study. J Gerontol A Biol Sci Med Sci. 2008;63:518–22.
13. McCorkle R, Strumpf NE, Nuamah IF, et al. A specialized home care intervention improves survival among older post-surgical cancer patients. J Am Geriatr Soc. 2000;48:1707–13.
14. Blanc-Bisson C, Fonck M, Rainfray M, et al. Undernutrition in elderly patients with cancer: target for diagnosis and intervention. Crit Rev Oncol Hematol. 2008;67:243–54.

15. Extermann M, Meyer J, McGinnis M, et al. A comprehensive geriatric intervention detects multiple problems in older breast cancer patients. Crit Rev Oncol Hematol. 2004;49:69–75.
16. Girre V, Falcou MC, Gisselbrecht M, et al. Does a geriatric oncology consultation modify the cancer treatment plan for elderly patients? J Gerontol A Biol Sci Med Sci. 2008;63:724–30.
17. Balducci L, Extermann M. Management of cancer in the older person: a practical approach. Oncologist. 2000;5:224–37.
18. Sanoff HK, Bleiberg H, Goldberg RM. Managing older patients with colorectal cancer. J Clin Oncol. 2007;25:1891–7.
19. Extermann M, Boler I, Reich RR, et al. Predicting the risk of chemotherapy toxicity in older patients: the Chemotherapy Risk Assessment Scale for High-Age Patients (CRASH) score. Cancer. 2012;118:3377–86.
20. Hutchins LF, Unger JM, Crowley JJ, et al. Underrepresentation of patients 65 years of age or older in cancer-treatment trials. N Engl J Med. 1999;341:2061–7.
21. Kemeny MM, Peterson BL, Kornblith AB, et al. Barriers to clinical trial participation by older women with breast cancer. J Clin Oncol. 2003;21:2268–75.
22. Mahoney T, Kuo YH, Topilow A, et al. Stage III colon cancers: why adjuvant chemotherapy is not offered to elderly patients. Arch Surg. 2000;135:182–5.
23. Extermann M, Albrand G, Chen H, et al. Are older French patients as willing as older American patients to undertake chemotherapy? J Clin Oncol. 2003;21:3214–9.
24. http://data.un.org/Data.aspx?d=GenderStat&f=inID%3A36. Accessed on December 4, 2012.
25. Sargent DJ, Patiyil S, Yothers G, et al. End points for colon cancer adjuvant trials: observations and recommendations based on individual patient data from 20,898 patients enrolled onto 18 randomized trials from the ACCENT Group. J Clin Oncol. 2007;25:4569–74.
26. Saltz LB, Niedzwiecki D, Hollis D, et al. Irinotecan fluorouracil plus leucovorin is not superior to fluorouracil plus leucovorin alone as adjuvant treatment for stage III colon cancer: results of CALGB 89803. J Clin Oncol. 2007;25:3456–61.
27. Van Cutsem E, Labianca R, Bodoky G, et al. Randomized phase III trial comparing biweekly infusional fluorouracil/leucovorin alone or with irinotecan in the adjuvant treatment of stage III colon cancer: PETACC-3. J Clin Oncol. 2009;27:3117–25.
28. Lembersky BC, Wieand HS, Petrelli NJ, et al. Oral uracil and tegafur plus leucovorin compared with intravenous fluorouracil and leucovorin in stage II and III carcinoma of the colon: results from National Surgical Adjuvant Breast and Bowel Project Protocol C-06. J Clin Oncol. 2006;24:2059–64.
29. Twelves C, Wong A, Nowacki MP, et al. Capecitabine as adjuvant treatment for stage III colon cancer. N Engl J Med. 2005;352:2696–704.
30. André T, Boni C, Navarro M, et al. Improved overall survival with oxaliplatin, fluorouracil, and leucovorin as adjuvant treatment in stage II or III colon cancer in the MOSAIC trial. J Clin Oncol. 2009;27:3109–16.
31. Haller DG, Tabernero J, Maroun J, et al. Capecitabine plus oxaliplatin compared with fluorouracil and folinic acid as adjuvant therapy for stage III colon cancer. J Clin Oncol. 2011;29:1465–71.
32. Tournigand C, de Gramont A. Chemotherapy: is adjuvant chemotherapy an option for stage II colon cancer? Nat Rev Clin Oncol. 2011;8:574–6.
33. Moertel CG, Fleming TR, Macdonald JS, et al. Levamisole and fluorouracil for adjuvant therapy of resected colon carcinoma. N Engl J Med. 1990;322:352–8.
34. Wolmark N, Rockette H, Mamounas E, et al. Clinical trial to assess the relative efficacy of fluorouracil and leucovorin, fluorouracil and levamisole, and fluorouracil, leucovorin, and levamisole in patients with Dukes' B and C carcinoma of the colon: results from National Surgical Adjuvant Breast and Bowel Project C-04. J Clin Oncol. 1999;17:3553–9.
35. André T, Quinaux E, Louvet C, et al. Phase III study comparing a semimonthly with a monthly regimen of fluorouracil and leucovorin as adjuvant treatment for stage II and III colon cancer patients: final results of GERCOR C96.1. J Clin Oncol. 2007;25:3732–8.
36. Gray R, Barnwell J, McConkey C, et al. Adjuvant chemotherapy versus observation in patients with colorectal cancer: a randomised study. Lancet. 2007;370:2020–9.

37. Sargent DJ, Marsoni S, Monges G, et al. Defective mismatch repair as a predictive marker for lack of efficacy of fluorouracil-based adjuvant therapy in colon cancer. J Clin Oncol. 2010;28: 3219–26.

38. André T. A multinational, randomized phase III study of bevacizumab with FOLFOX4 or XELOX versus FOLFOX4 alone as adjuvant treatment for colon cancer: subgroup analyses from the AVANT trial. J Clin Oncol. 2011;29:223s.

39. Alberts SR, Sargent DJ, Smyrrk TC, et al. Adjuvant mFOLFOX6 with or without cetuximab in KRAS wild-type patients with resected stage III colon cancer: results from NCCTG intergroup phase III trial N0147. J Clin Oncol. 2010;28:959s.

40. Allegra CJ, Yothers G, O'Connell MJ, et al. Phase III trial assessing bevacizumab in stages II and III carcinoma of the colon: results of NSABP protocol C-08. J Clin Oncol. 2011;29: 11–6.

41. Sargent DJ, Goldberg RM, Jacobson SD, et al. A pooled analysis of adjuvant chemotherapy for resected colon cancer in elderly patients. N Engl J Med. 2001;345:1091–7.

42. Iwashyna TJ, Lamont EB. Effectiveness of adjuvant fluorouracil in clinical practice: a population-based cohort study of elderly patients with stage III colon cancer. J Clin Oncol. 2002;20:3992–8.

43. Kahn KL, Adams JL, Weeks JC, et al. Adjuvant chemotherapy use and adverse events among older patients with stage III colon cancer. JAMA. 2010;303:1037–45.

44. Jackson McCleary NA, Meyerhardt J, Green E, et al. Impact of older age on the efficacy of newer adjuvant therapies in >12500 patients with stage II/III colon cancer: findings from the ACCENT database. J Clin Oncol. 2009;27(15S):4010.

45. Tournigand C, André T, Bonnetain F, et al. Adjuvant therapy with 5-fluorouracil and oxaliplatin in stage II and elderly patients (aged between 70 and 75 years) with colon cancer: subgroup analyses of the MOSAIC Trial. J Clin Oncol. 2012;30(27):3353–60.

46. Haller D, Cassidy J, Tabernero J, et al. Phase III trial of capecitabine + oxaliplatin vs bolus 5-FU/LV in stage III colon cancer (NO16968): impact of age on DFS and OS. ASCO GI, San Fransico, 2010

47. Yothers G, O'Connell MJ, Allegra CJ, et al. Oxaliplatin as adjuvant therapy for colon cancer: updated results of NSABP C-07 trial, including survival and subset analyses. J Clin Oncol. 2011;29:3768–74.

48. Haller DG, O'Connell M, Cartwright TH, et al. Impact of age and medical comorbidity (MC) on adjuvant treatment outcomes for stage III colon cancer (CC): a pooled analysis of individual patient data from four randomized controlled trials. J Clin Oncol. 2012;30(suppl; abstr 3522).

49. Saliba D, Elliott M, Rubenstein LZ, et al. The Vulnerable Elders Survey: a tool for identifying vulnerable older people in the community. J Am Geriatr Soc. 2001;49:1691–9.

50. Luciani A, Ascione G, Bertuzzi C, et al. Detecting disabilities in older patients with cancer: comparison between comprehensive geriatric assessment and vulnerable elders survey-13. J Clin Oncol. 2010;28:2046–50.

51. Goldberg RM, Tabah-Fisch I, Bleiberg H, et al. Pooled analysis of safety and efficacy of oxaliplatin plus fluorouracil/leucovorin administered bimonthly in elderly patients with colorectal cancer. J Clin Oncol. 2006;24:4085–91.

52. Schmoll HJ, Cartwright T, Tabernero J, et al. Phase III trial of capecitabine plus oxaliplatin as adjuvant therapy for stage III colon cancer: a planned safety analysis in 1,864 patients. J Clin Oncol. 2007;25:102–9.

53. Feliu J, Escudero P, Llosa F, et al. Capecitabine as first-line treatment for patients older than 70 years with metastatic colorectal cancer: an oncopaz cooperative group study. J Clin Oncol. 2005;23:3104–11.

54. Feliu J, Salud A, Escudero P, et al. XELOX (capecitabine plus oxaliplatin) as first-line treatment for elderly patients over 70 years of age with advanced colorectal cancer. Br J Cancer. 2006;94:969–75.

55. de Gramont A, Chibaudel B, Bachet JB, et al. From chemotherapy to targeted therapy in adjuvant treatment for stage III colon cancer. Semin Oncol. 2011;38:521–32.

56. Buyse M, Sargent DJ, Grothey A, et al. Biomarkers and surrogate end points – the challenge of statistical validation. Nat Rev Clin Oncol. 2010;7:309–17.
57. Gray RG, Quirke P, Handley K, et al. Validation study of a quantitative multigene reverse transcriptase-polymerase chain reaction assay for assessment of recurrence risk in patients with stage II colon cancer. J Clin Oncol. 2011;29:4611–9.
58. Kennedy RD, Bylesjo M, Kerr P, et al. Development and independent validation of a prognostic assay for stage II colon cancer using formalin-fixed paraffin-embedded tissue. J Clin Oncol. 2011;29:4620–6.

Chapter 11
Chemotherapy in the Metastatic Setting

Gunnar Folprecht

Abstract Balancing between the competing risks of tumor death and toxicity with the influence of comorbidity and ageing on both, prognosis and treatment tolerability are essential for treatment decisions in elderly patients.

For patients enrolled in clinical trials, meta-analyses have shown an efficacy of chemotherapy in elderly patients similar to younger patients and no major differences in treatment effect. Nonrandomized phase II trials in elderly patients demonstrated similar results with chemotherapy as for younger patients. These analyses have therefore the methodological problem that the age distribution in clinical trials does not reflect daily clinical practice and that only a subset of elderly patients participated in the trials. The British FOCUS 2 enrolling frail patients demonstrated a better "overall treatment utility" if patients were treated with combination chemotherapy instead of fluoropyrimidine monotherapy.

Keywords Metastatic colorectal cancer • Elderly patients • Chemotherapy • 5-FU • Fluoropyrimidine • Oxaliplatin • Irinotecan • Comorbidity • Stage IV metastases • Palliative chemotherapy

Introduction

During the last decades, major advances were achieved in the treatment of patients with metastatic colorectal cancer. 5-Fluorouracil and its oral prodrugs are still some of the most important drugs in colorectal cancer, although the efficacy of systemic treatment was improved when further cytotoxic drugs (irinotecan and oxaliplatin)

G. Folprecht, Ph.D.
Medical Department I/University Cancer Center, University Hospital
Carl Gustav Carus, Fetscherstr. 74, Dresden 01307, Germany
e-mail: gunnar.folprecht@uniklinikum-dresden.de

D. Papamichael, R.A. Audisio (eds.), *Management of Colorectal Cancers in Older People*,   129
DOI 10.1007/978-0-85729-984-0_11, © Springer-Verlag London 2013

were introduced. Monoclonal antibodies targeting the vascular endothelial growth factor (VEGF) and the epidermal growth factor receptor (EGFR) further increased survival in patients with metastatic colorectal cancer. Most recently, studies have shown prolongation of survival when pretreated patients received the fusion protein aflibercept [1] or the multi-kinase inhibitor regorafenib [2]. At least for the use of EGFR antibodies, molecular tumor characteristics (k-ras and b-raf) can define subgroups with higher probability for response to treatment. Despite these advances in "targeted therapies" – the special aspects of which related to geriatric patients are discussed in Chap. 12 – chemotherapy remains the mainstay of treatment in metastatic colorectal cancer.

Balancing between the competing risks of tumor death and toxicity with the influence of comorbidity and ageing on both, prognosis and treatment tolerability are essential for treatment decisions in elderly patients. As for many tumor types, the age distribution in clinical trials does not reflect what happens in everyday clinical practice. Exclusion criteria of the trials, age limits within the trials, or medical/social conditions regarded by the treating physician as a contraindication to treatment contribute to this situation. An age-dependent referral bias to clinical trial centers may additionally contribute to a highly selected patient population.

Meta-analyses of General Studies in Colorectal Cancer

For patients enrolled in clinical trials, meta-analyses have shown an efficacy of chemotherapy in elderly patients similar to younger patients and no major differences in treatment effect. The main methodological problem is that only a subset of elderly patients – fulfilling the inclusion criteria and actually enrolled by the treating physician – participated in the trials and could be subject of these analyses. Due to the limited number of randomized trials focusing on the elderly, these analyses can only be informative for treatment decisions in elderly patients with good performance status and limited comorbidities.

In an analysis of 3,825 patients treated with 5-FU/FA in 22 trials, there was no difference in response to chemotherapy or overall survival. The progression-free survival was statistically significantly longer in elderly patients with an age ≥70 years, but the difference was not clinically relevant. Data on treatment-associated toxicity are not available; the 60-day mortality as an indicator for severe early toxicity did not differ between the two age groups (Table 11.1) [3].

For oxaliplatin-based therapy, there is one larger analysis available including one first-line trial of FOLFOX versus IFL and three trials comparing FOLFOX to 5-FU/FA in the adjuvant, first-, or second-line treatment, respectively. In the pooled analysis, there was no interaction between age and treatment regarding PFS/DFS and OS. In total, there were 1,496 patients receiving first- or second-line treatment in metastatic colorectal cancer enrolled. In the three trials in the metastatic setting, no significant interaction between age and response rate was

Table 11.1 Pooled analyses from randomized trials investigating chemotherapy in metastatic colorectal cancer

	N	Patients ≥70 years	Elderly patients (≥70 years)			Younger patients (<70 years)		
			RR	PFS months, 95 % CI	OS months, 95 % CI	RR	PFS months, 95 % CI	OS months, 95 % CI
5-FU/FA 1st line [3]	3,825	629	23.9 %	5.3 (5.2–5.8)	10.8 (9.7–11.8)	21.1 %	5.3 (5.1–5.5)	11.3 (10.9–11.7)
Bolus[a]	2,527	456	21.3 %	5.2 (4.4–5.9)	10.3 (9.0–11.5)	18.5 %	4.8 (4.5–5.1)	10.8 (10.3–11.2)
Infusion[a]	1,297	173	31.2 %	5.8 (4.2–7.4)	11.9 (9.4–14.5)	26.2 %	5.9 (5.5–6.2)	12.3 (11.5–13.2)
Irinotecan/5-FU 1st line [4]	2,691	599						
Irinotecan/5-FU/FA	997	220	50.5 % (43.5–57.5)	9.2 (8.0–10.4)	14.5 (11.1–17.9)	46.6 % (42.9–50.2)	8.2 (7.7–8.7)	17.1 (15.9–18.3)
5-FU/FA	1,694	379	30.3 % (25.5–35.5)	7.7 (6.1–9.3)	14.2 (10.8–17.7)	29.0 % (26.4–31.6)	6.3 (5.9–6.7)	14.7 (13.9–15.6)
FOLFOX diff. lines [5]	3,742 (meta-static: 1496)	614 (metastatic: 299)	NR	HR 0.70 (95 % CI 0.63–0.77)	HR 0.77 (95 % CI 0.67–0.88)	NR	HR 0.65 (95 % CI 0.52–0.81)	HR 0.82 (95 % CI 0.63–1.06)

[a]Most trials were not designed to compare 5-FU infusion to 5-FU bolus application

Table 11.2 Age groups in meta-analyses from clinical trials investigating chemotherapy in metastatic colorectal cancer

	Oxaliplatin/5-FU/FA (metastatic patients) [5]	Fluoropyrimidines [3]	Irinotecan/5-FU/FA [4]
All pts	1,496 (100 %)	3,825 (100 %)	2,691 (100 %)
≥70	299 (20.0 %)	629 (22.3 %)	599 (16.4 %)
≥75	118 (7.9 %)	145 (3.8 %)	185 (5.4 %)
≥80	18 (1.2 %)	20 (0.5 %)	25 (0.9 %)

observed (Table 11.1) [5]. In four studies comparing the combination of irinotecan plus 5-FU/FA and 5-FU/FA monotherapy in the first-line therapy of metastatic colorectal cancer (2,691 patients), the treatment effect was generally not age dependent (Table 11.1). Interestingly, in the subgroup of patients treated with the more toxic IFL (irinotecan/bolus 5-FU) regimen, the survival of elderly patients has shown a trend to be worse than with 5-FU alone. Furthermore, in patients with ≥75 years, there was no clear benefit for combination therapy. While this subgroup analysis is limited by the relatively small number of patients (185 patients were ≥75 years old), it represents one of the largest randomized comparisons in this age group, and it should be noted that the patients are – as in most clinical trials – highly selected [4].

The cutoff in all cited combined analyses was 70 years, but patients ≥75 represent only 5–6 % of the entire trial populations, and patients ≥80 years were rare (~1 %, Table 11.2) [3–5]. Because the analyses for "elderly" patients (≥70 years) are mainly influenced by the age group of 70–75, it remains uncertain as to whether the results for elderly patients can be generalized to the majority of patients over 75 and especially over 80 years (Table 11.2).

With FOLFOX treatment, significantly more grade 3/4 neutropenia and thrombocytopenia were reported in elderly patients (49 % vs. 43 %, 5 % vs. 2 %). In addition, increased fatigue and decreased nausea/vomiting were associated with increasing age as a continuous variable demonstrating that there was no clear age cutoff for these two toxicities [5]. Less vomiting/nausea was found for elderly patients treated with 5-FU/FA monotherapy in the irinotecan trials, too. With irinotecan combinations, there was a significant influence of age as a continuous variable (not with the cutoff of 70 years) on the frequency of diarrhea [4].

A combined analysis for capecitabine described gastrointestinal toxicity in particular as being increased in patients with higher age. In a univariate analysis, both age and renal function (creatinine clearance) correlated with toxicity. In the multivariate analysis, renal function only remained with significant influence. The authors explained this effect with higher exposure to the 5-FU precursor 5′-DFUR being increased in patients with impaired renal function. However, the same effect of higher toxicity was observed in patients treated with bolus 5-FU/FA as in the Mayo Clinic regimen in the same trials [6] – without the 5-FU precursor. A correlation of decreased creatinine clearance with other factors/comorbidities would be another explanation, and creatinine clearance was associated in later analyses of general chemotherapy toxicity with higher toxicity [7]. Reduced starting doses for capecitabine are recommended for patients with moderately decreased creatinine clearance (30–50 ml/min).

Age-dependent dosing was recommended for irinotecan as monotherapy per prescription information (300 instead of 350 mg/m^2) together with reduction for other factors such as previous pelvic irradiation by the manufacturer. Chau and colleagues analyzed a trial which used the full dose of irinotecan in younger and elderly patients. In total, 339 patients were enrolled; 72 patients were ≥70 years. The investigators found more neutropenia in elderly patients. The toxicity according to a combined endpoint of grade 3/4 diarrhea, nausea/vomiting, and fever/infection was not increased. Efficacy was similar in both age groups [8].

Trials in Elderly Patients

The British FOCUS 2 trial enrolled patients who were – according to the opinion of the treating physician – not candidates for full dose chemotherapy [9]. In a 2 × 2 factorial design, substitution of 5-FU by capecitabine and combination therapy with oxaliplatin ("XELOX" or FOLFOX schedules) versus fluoropyrimidine monotherapy were tested. The inclusion criterion of performance status did not differ from the FOCUS trial (WHO PS 0–2), but the creatinine clearance could be lower (≥30 instead of ≥50 ml/min), and inclusion criteria were more liberal with regard to other laboratory parameters (bilirubin ≤3 × ULN instead of ≤1.25 × ULN, thrombocytes ≥100 instead of ≥150 Gpt/l, white blood count ≥3.0 instead of ≥4.0 Gpt/l), but there was no special selection for geriatric patients. Although the median age in the FOCUS 2 trial is higher (74 years) than in the FOCUS trial (64 years), it is with an age range of 35–87 years, not a trial purely performed in geriatric patients. One quarter of patients were younger than 70 years.

The dose recommended per protocol in the FOCUS2 trial was 80 % of the standard dose. When the creatinine clearance was <50 ml/min, oxaliplatin and capecitabine were further reduced by 25 %. An advantage of substituting infusional 5-FU by capecitabine could not be demonstrated; on the contrary, there was significantly more toxicity with capecitabine, especially more nausea, vomiting, anorexia grade 2, more diarrhea grades 2 and 3, and more hand-foot syndrome. Interestingly, the addition of oxaliplatin did not increase the overall frequency of toxicity but of some items.

There was a significantly better response rate with oxaliplatin-based therapy (35 % vs. 15 %, $p < 0.0001$) and a trend toward longer progression-free survival with the oxaliplatin combination (HR 0.84, 95 % CI 0.69–1.01, $p=0.07$). All other classical efficacy parameters did not show a difference.

The authors defined an innovative composite endpoint of "overall treatment utility" (OTU) after 12 weeks. Overall treatment utility was "good" if there was no clinical or radiological evidence of progression, there were no major negative effects in terms of toxicity, and the patient's own assessment was that the treatment was worthwhile. A "good" outcome was more probable with oxaliplatin (47 % vs. 36 %, $p<0.003$), but not with capecitabine (44 % vs. 39 %). Better baseline EQ5D, baseline overall symptom score, Nottingham ADL, WBC ≤10 Gpt/l, and albumin ≥30 g/l were associated with "good" treatment outcome. Interestingly, only 14 % of patients did not have a dose reduction, justifying the planned up-front dose reduction.

The French FFCD group presented interims results of a trial enrolling patients ≥75 years [10]. Two hundred and nine patients were randomized to 5-FU/FA with or without irinotecan, and 166 patients were included in the interim analysis. The median age of patients in the trial was 80 years. Comorbidity in these patients was relatively low; the majority had a Charlson comorbidity index of zero, nearly all patients ≤2. However, the 60-day mortality rate in these patients was 12.7 %, although the investigators regarded two deaths as related to treatment only. Response to treatment was higher in patients treated with combination therapy; toxicity (diarrhea, nausea/vomiting, asthenia), too. The results of the more relevant time-dependent endpoints are not yet available.

When the data of the FOCUS 2 trial [9] and the FFCD trial [10] are compared to data in general trials with predominantly younger population, the academic trials from the same study groups (FOCUS and FFCD 2000–05) [11, 12] comparing up-front combination therapy to the sequential use of 5-FU followed by combination therapy or up-front combination therapy should be considered. In these trials, differences in overall survival could not be demonstrated (FFCD) or were very small (FOCUS) – even in a population with better treatment tolerability for combination therapy. Despite the results of these trials and other studies investigating combination versus sequential treatment [13], combination therapy is mostly regarded as standard and has widespread use. The main reason is that most registration and other earlier trials have demonstrated a survival benefit for the combination therapy. In a pooled analysis from these earlier trials in the general patient population, patients with a performance status 2 derive the same benefit from combination therapy as patients with better performance status, but they have an increased 60-day mortality (12 % in PS 2 vs. 3 % in PS 0–1 patients) [14]. In contrast to the general trial population, comorbidity instead of tumor symptoms is more likely to contribute to the reduced performance status in elderly patients. Therefore, the results of the general (younger) trial population with decreased performance status cannot be applied to elderly patients without restrictions. Nevertheless, combination therapy was also recommended by the FOCUS 2 authors as a result of their trial due to the better "overall treatment utility" in the composite endpoint as discussed above [9].

Numerous small phase II trials were conducted in more or less elderly patients (Table 11.3). Unfortunately, the generally small number of patients and the lack of an internal control limit the value for further treatment decisions. When the inclusion criteria are reviewed, it becomes obvious that they do not differ markedly from trials in the general population of patients with metastatic colorectal cancer. All trials excluded patients with a performance status <2, some trials even patients with a performance status of one. Patients with more severe comorbidities were excluded in virtually all trials. Although most studies enrolled patients with an age of ≥70 or ≥72, the median age was 75–76, and a small minority had an age >80 years, only. Not surprisingly with regard to the inclusion criteria, most patients had few comorbidities. As a result, the outcomes are similar to the subgroup analyses known from the phase III trials. It is within this line that most of these trials did not identify problems in terms of administering the drugs in full doses. With the small number of patients, subgroup analyses regarding comorbidity, IADL, or ADL did not produce significant results, even where a geriatric assessment was reported. Two conclusions can be drawn from this situation. Firstly, trials focusing on patients who are more frail do not fulfill the inclusion criteria for standard clinical trials. Inclusion of patients over 80 could perhaps answer more outstanding questions for clinical practice. The EORTC is launching such a clinical trial focusing on patients with severe comorbidity or an age ≥80 years. Secondly, standardized geriatric baseline evaluation and reporting of elderly trials according to these baseline characteristics would increase the chances of comparing different phase II trials in the absence of randomized comparisons and might potentially better define which patients do not derive benefit from a given (full dose) therapy.

Such trials outside the standard trial population require more open inclusion criteria and will be conducted in situations that are usually defined as contraindication to the drug. To overcome the safety aspects, dose-reduced schedules might be a useful option as demonstrated by the FOCUS investigators. To investigate these situations in clinical trials is urgently needed as daily practice requires treatment decisions even if patients have abnormal laboratory values and some comorbidity or the physician is uncertain whether they can tolerate chemotherapy.

With the limitation that the data are mainly generated in diseases other than colorectal cancer, some estimates for chemotherapy toxicity beyond the geriatric assessment may be helpful. The CRASH score (www.moffitt.org/saoptools; accessed July 25, 2012) calculates increased risk of hematologic toxicity with diastolic blood pressure (>72), IADL (<26), LDH (>0.74*ULN), non-hematologic toxicity performance status (>0), mini mental health status (<30), and minimal nutritional assessment (<28). The chemotherapy regimen is considered in both scores as an additional risk factor. This score was developed in 331 patients and validated in 187 patients – 12 % had colorectal cancer and 55 % of all patients were in stage IV – and allows to discriminate the risk of hematologic toxicity of <10 % in the lowest-risk group to >90 % in the highest-risk group, for non-hematologic toxicity from <40 to >90 % [25].

Another risk score was developed by Hurria and colleagues and was shown to be superior to the physician-estimated Karnofsky performance status [7]. They proposed

Table 11.3 Phase II studies – chemotherapy in elderly patients with metastatic CRC

Authors	n	Inclusion criteria	Treatment	RR	PFS (months)	OS (months)	Comorbidity/(I) ADL
Feliu et al. [15]	38	≥70 years	UFT/FA	29 %	NR	NR	Charlson
Feliu et al. [16]	51	≥70 years	Capecitabine	24 %	7	11	0 – 80 %
		PS ≤2	2 × 1,250				1 – 16 %
		Not suitable for combination					2 – 4 %
							Dose intensity 88 %
Mattioli et al. [17]	78	≥70 years	FOLFOX split to d1/2	51 %	8	20	ADL at baseline 5.7
		PS ≤2					IADL 4.2
Rosati et al. [18]	47	≥70 years PS ≤2	UFT/FA/OX	51 %	8	14.1	ADL score
							6 – 43 %
							5 – 11 %
							4 – 6 %
							≤3 – 19 %
							NA – 19 %
							IADL
							100 – 19 %
							75–99 – 26 %
							<75 – 36 %
							NA – 19 %
Rosati et al. [19]	47	≥70 years PS ≤2	CapIri	36 %	7	14.0	
	47		CapOx	38 %	8	19.3	

Reference	N	Inclusion criteria	Regimen				Comments
Comella et al. [20]	76	≥70 years PS ≤2 Minimal mental ≥26 Charlson ≤4	XELOX	41	8.5	14.4	Charlson 0 – 36 % 1 – 40 % 2 – 16 % ≥3 – 8 %
Feliu et al. [21]	50	≥70 years PS ≤2	XELOX	36	58	13.2	Charlson 0 – 60 % 1 – 26 % 2 – 8 % 3 – 6 % Dose intensity 86–98 %
Benavides et al. [22]	129	≥70 years PS ≤2	Oxaliplatin/5-FU [48 h]	52	9.1	16.3	Comorbidity listing not standardized (i.e., benign prostate hypertrophy)
Souglakos et al. [23]	30	≥70 years PS ≤2	FOLFIRI	37	7	14.5	
Sastre et al. [24]	85	≥72 years PS ≤1	Irinotecan/5-FU[48 h]	35	8	15.3	

three scores for hemoglobin <11/10 g/l (male/female patients), creatinine clearance <34 ml/min, and one or more falls in the last 6 months; two scores for age ≥72 years, gastrointestinal or genitourinary cancer, polychemotherapy, hearing loss (fair/worse), and walking limited to <1 block; and one score for taking medications with help/unable to take medications (IADL) and at least sometimes decreased social activity because of physical/emotional health. With ≤5 scores, the risk for grade ≥3 toxicity is 30 %, with 6–9 scores 52 %, and with ≥10 scores 83 %. In contrast, the physician-rated Karnofsky performance status did not significantly discriminate the probability for toxicity (PS ≥90 %, risk of grade ≥3 toxicity 51 %; PS 80 %, risk of toxicity 51 %; ≤70 %, risk of toxicity 62 %). An open question is the best treatment for patients with increased risk for toxicity.

Until more results from clinical trials are available, it can be concluded that patients with limited comorbidities and good performance status (or low risk for toxicity) can be treated with the same regimens as younger patients. Experiences from the IFL regimen discussed above demonstrate that avoiding high toxicity may be still important even in the elderly clinical trial population. For frail patients, the FOCUS 2 trial has demonstrated that capecitabine but not dose-reduced combination increased toxicity and that the combination therapy with infusional 5-FU (including dose reductions) has provided the best overall treatment outcome. As the results with irinotecan are similar in all other situations, irinotecan per se should not be excluded in this group of patients. Probably, the results for frail patients can be generalized to patients >80 years, but the clinical trial experience in this age group is astonishingly limited given that colorectal cancer is one of the most common type of cancers.

References

1. Van Cutsem E, Tabernero J, Lakomy R, et al. Intravenous (iv) aflibercept versus placebo in combination with irinotecan/5-fu (FOLFIRI) for second-line treatment of metastatic colorectal cancer (mCRC): results of a multinational phase III trial (EFC10262-VELOUR). Ann Oncol. 2011;22(5s; abstr O-0024).
2. Grothey A, Sobrero A, Siena S, et al. Results of a phase III randomized, double-blind, placebo-controlled, multicenter trial (CORRECT) of regorafenib plus best supportive care (BSC) versus placebo plus BSC in patients (pts) with metastatic colorectal cancer (mCRC) who have progressed after standard therapies. J Clin Oncol. 2012; 30(suppl 4; abstr LBA385).
3. Folprecht G, Cunningham D, Ross P, et al. Efficacy of 5-fluorouracil-based chemotherapy in elderly patients with metastatic colorectal cancer: a pooled analysis of clinical trials. Ann Oncol. 2004;15(9):1330–8.
4. Folprecht G, Seymour MT, Saltz L, et al. Irinotecan/fluorouracil combination in first-line therapy of older and younger patients with metastatic colorectal cancer: combined analysis of 2,691 patients in randomized controlled trials. J Clin Oncol. 2008;26(9):1443–51.
5. Goldberg RM, Tabah-Fisch I, Bleiberg H, et al. Pooled analysis of safety and efficacy of oxaliplatin plus fluorouracil/leucovorin administered bimonthly in elderly patients with colorectal cancer. J Clin Oncol. 2006;24(25):4085–91.
6. Cassidy J, Twelves C, Van Cutsem E, et al. First-line oral capecitabine therapy in metastatic colorectal cancer: a favorable safety profile compared with intravenous 5-fluorouracil/leucovorin. Ann Oncol. 2002;13(4):566–75.

7. Hurria A, Togawa K, Mohile SG, et al. Predicting chemotherapy toxicity in older adults with cancer: a prospective multicenter study. J Clin Oncol. 2011;29(25):3457–65.
8. Chau I, Norman AR, Cunningham D, et al. Elderly patients with fluoropyrimidine and thymidylate synthase inhibitor-resistant advanced colorectal cancer derive similar benefit without excessive toxicity when treated with irinotecan monotherapy. Br J Cancer. 2004;91(8):1453–8.
9. Seymour M. Sequential chemotherapy for colorectal cancer. Lancet Oncol. 2011;12(11):987–8.
10. Mitry E, Phelip F, Bonnetain F, et al. Phase III trial of chemotherapy with or without irinotecan in the front-line treatment of metastatic colorectal cancer in elderly patients (FFCD 2001–02 trial): results of a planned interim analysis. In: Proceedings of gastrointestinal cancer symposium (ASCO/AGA/ASTRO/SSO). 2008. Abstract 281.
11. Seymour MT, Maughan TS, Ledermann JA, et al. Different strategies of sequential and combination chemotherapy for patients with poor prognosis advanced colorectal cancer (MRC FOCUS): a randomised controlled trial. Lancet. 2007;370(9582):143–52.
12. Ducreux M, Malka D, Mendiboure J, et al. Sequential versus combination chemotherapy for the treatment of advanced colorectal cancer (FFCD 2000–05): an open-label, randomised, phase 3 trial. Lancet Oncol. 2011;12(11):1032–44.
13. Koopman M, Antonini NF, Douma J, et al. Sequential versus combination chemotherapy with capecitabine, irinotecan, and oxaliplatin in advanced colorectal cancer (CAIRO): a phase III randomised controlled trial. Lancet. 2007;370(9582):135–42.
14. Sargent DJ, Kohne CH, Sanoff HK, et al. Pooled safety and efficacy analysis examining the effect of performance status on outcomes in nine first-line treatment trials using individual data from patients with metastatic colorectal cancer. J Clin Oncol. 2009;27(12):1948–55.
15. Feliu J, Gonzalez BM, Espinosa E, et al. Uracil and tegafur modulated with leucovorin: an effective regimen with low toxicity for the treatment of colorectal carcinoma in the elderly. Oncopaz Cooperative Group. Cancer. 1997;79(10):1884–9.
16. Feliu J, Escudero P, Llosa F, et al. Capecitabine as first-line treatment for patients older than 70 years with metastatic colorectal cancer: an oncopaz cooperative group study. J Clin Oncol. 2005;23(13):3104–11.
17. Mattioli R, Massacesi C, Recchia F, et al. High activity and reduced neurotoxicity of bi-fractionated oxaliplatin plus 5-fluorouracil/leucovorin for elderly patients with advanced colorectal cancer. Ann Oncol. 2005;16(7):1147–51.
18. Rosati G, Cordio S, Tucci A, et al. Phase II trial of oxaliplatin and tegafur/uracil and oral folinic acid for advanced or metastatic colorectal cancer in elderly patients. Oncology. 2005;69(2):122–9.
19. Rosati G, Cordio S, Bordonaro R, et al. Capecitabine in combination with oxaliplatin or irinotecan in elderly patients with advanced colorectal cancer: results of a randomized phase II study. Ann Oncol. 2010;21(4):781–6.
20. Comella P, Natale D, Farris A, et al. Capecitabine plus oxaliplatin for the first-line treatment of elderly patients with metastatic colorectal carcinoma: final results of the Southern Italy Cooperative Oncology Group Trial 0108. Cancer. 2005;104(2):282–9.
21. Feliu J, Salud A, Escudero P, et al. XELOX (capecitabine plus oxaliplatin) as first-line treatment for elderly patients over 70 years of age with advanced colorectal cancer. Br J Cancer. 2006;94(7):969–75.
22. Benavides M, Pericay C, Valladares-Ayerbes M, et al. Oxaliplatin in combination with infusional 5-fluorouracil as first-line chemotherapy for elderly patients with metastatic colorectal cancer: a phase II study of the Spanish Cooperative Group for the Treatment of Digestive Tumors. Clin Colorectal Cancer. 2012;11:200–6.
23. Souglakos J, Pallis A, Kakolyris S, et al. Combination of irinotecan (CPT-11) plus 5-fluorouracil and leucovorin (FOLFIRI regimen) as first line treatment for elderly patients with metastatic colorectal cancer: a phase II trial. Oncology. 2005;69(5):384–90.
24. Sastre J, Marcuello E, Masutti B, et al. Irinotecan in combination with fluorouracil in a 48-hour continuous infusion as first-line chemotherapy for elderly patients with metastatic colorectal cancer: a Spanish cooperative group for the treatment of digestive tumors study. J Clin Oncol. 2005;23(15):3545–51.
25. Extermann M, Boler I, Reich RR, et al. Predicting the risk of chemotherapy toxicity in older patients: the Chemotherapy Risk Assessment Scale for High-Age Patients (CRASH) score. Cancer. 2012;118(13):3377–86.

Chapter 12
Targeted Therapies in Older Patients with Metastatic Colorectal Cancer

Javier Sastre, Jon Zugazagoitia, Aranzazu Manzano, and Eduardo Díaz-Rubio

Abstract During the last years, targeted therapies have been incorporated to the treatment of patients with metastatic colorectal cancer. Whereas the main pivotal or registry studies of these drugs did not systematically exclude elderly people, they formed a minority of these cohorts. Data from studies nonselected by age and age-selected suggest that age alone should not be an exclusion criterion for receiving bevacizumab plus CT in mCRC. Fit elderly patients derive similar benefit in terms of RR, PFS, and OS with the use of bevacizumab plus CT. All studies are consistent in establishing that elderly patients have an increased incidence of ATEs with respect to younger ones, and therefore, those with a recent episode of myocardial infarction, stroke, or any other arterial thrombotic event should be excluded from receiving bevacizumab. Cetuximab and panitumumab seem to have a similar safety profile in the elderly compared to younger patients, either as single agent or in combination with CT. Thus, age alone should not be a condition to exclude the use of these drugs in the mCRC treatment setting.

Keywords Metastatic • Colorectal • Older patients • Monoclonal antibodies • Elderly patients • Colorectal cancer • Bevacizumab • EGFR inhibitors • Targeted therapies

J. Sastre, Ph.D. (✉)
Gastrointestinal Unit, Oncology Department, HC San Carlos,
Martin Lagos, Madrid 28040, Spain
e-mail: jsastre.hcsc@salud.madrid.org

J. Zugazagoitia, M.D. • A. Manzano, M.D. • E. Díaz-Rubio, Ph.D.
Oncology Department, HC San Carlos,
Martin Lagos, Madrid 28040, Spain

D. Papamichael, R.A. Audisio (eds.), *Management of Colorectal Cancers in Older People*, 141
DOI 10.1007/978-0-85729-984-0_12, © Springer-Verlag London 2013

Introduction

Monoclonal antibodies against specific molecular targets such as vascular endothe-lial growth factor (VEGF) or epidermal growth factor receptor (EGFR) have meant a breakthrough in the treatment of metastatic colorectal cancer (mCRC), allowing to optimize the results achieved with conventional chemotherapy (CT). Whereas the main pivotal or registry studies of these drugs did not systematically exclude elderly people, they formed a minority of these cohorts. Moreover, elderly participants in these trials usually are carefully selected specially with regard to low comorbidity, so they are not always representative of the overall elderly population. On the other hand, there are only few studies testing the safety and efficacy of biologic targeted agents exclusively in elderly patients. However, selecting old people exclusively based on chronologic age has some limitations, due to the heterogeneity inherent to older people mainly in relation to comorbidity, functional status, and mental health among others [1, 2]. These studies selected by age not always had homogeneous criteria to select well-defined elderly cohorts based on all these aspects, making it difficult to integrate findings into daily clinical practice. In this chapter, we will analyze separately the results of elderly patients included in studies nonselected by age and those which exclusively included a defined elderly cohort.

Bevacizumab

The role of angiogenesis in tumor growth and metastasis is apparent from the high density of vasculature observed in large tumors. VEGF is the most important media-tor of the angiogenic process. In many tumor types, VEGF expression is upregu-lated, and it has been shown as a prognostic factor [3]. The humanized monoclonal antibody bevacizumab (Avastin®), which is the only antiangiogenic agent approved for colorectal cancer treatment, was shown to produce important changes on tumor vasculature leading to a lower density and interstitial pressure. This vascular nor-malization can alleviate hypoxia and make drug delivery more efficient. Due to this mechanism of action, its lack of activity against tumor growth in vitro, and the syn-ergistic effect together with cytotoxic agents in human cells lines in animal models, bevacizumab has been developed in association with chemotherapy.

Studies Nonselected by Age

Analysis of Randomized Controlled Trials (RCT)

In the first registry study in first-line treatment of advanced disease (AVF2107), the addition of bevacizumab to a standard irinotecan + 5-FU/LV regimen demonstrated prolonged overall survival (OS) of almost 5 months. Patient accrual was not restricted by age, and the subgroup of patients aged >65 years (32 % of the entire cohort) obtained similar benefits from bevacizumab therapy compared to the overall population [4].

Currently, we have two pooled analyses of the elderly patients included in the main RCT with bevacizumab in mCRC [5, 6]. The first one was published by Kabbinavar et al. and analyzed a total of 439 patients ≥65 years old who had been previously included in two of the pivotal studies in first-line therapy, the previously mentioned AVF2107 (IFL ± bevacizumab) and AVF2192 [7] (5-FU/LV ± bevacizumab) trials. In addition to the CT regimen used in combination with bevacizumab, both studies were markedly different with regard to patients baseline demographics, since, among other differences, the AVF2192 study was composed exclusively of patients not considered candidates for irinotecan therapy. Due to this fact, a categorical variable was used to adjust for these differences. Of these 439 patients, 218 received CT+bevacizumab and 221 CT+placebo. The benefit of adding bevacizumab to CT compared to placebo+CT in the ≥65-year-old cohort was comparable to what is observed for the overall AVF2107 population, both in OS (19.3 vs. 14.3 months, respectively, HR 0.70, IC 95 % 0.55–0.90, $p=0.006$) as progression-free survival (PFS) (9.2 vs. 6.2 months, respectively, HR 0.52, IC 95 % 0.40–0.67, $p<0.0001$). In addition, similar results were found in an exploratory analysis of 276 patients ≥70 years old. With regard to toxicity, among the grade (G) 3–4 adverse events related with bevacizumab, significantly higher rates of hypertension was found in this patient subgroup (13.8 vs. 1.8 % for patients treated with and without bevacizumab, respectively). Likewise, the incidence of arterial thromboembolic events (ATEs) was 2.5 times higher in patients treated with bevacizumab in this population, without significant differences in venous thromboembolic events (VTEs) [5].

More recently, Cassidy et al. conducted a second pooled analysis with a greater number of patients in order to compare differences in terms of efficacy and safety of CT+bevacizumab between older and younger patients (unlike the one published by Kabbinavar et al. where a formal comparison between both age groups was not carried out). For this analysis, the four major RCT with bevacizumab in mCRC were included, three in first-line therapy (AVF2107, AVF2192 and NO16966 [8]) and one in second-line (E3200) [9]. In these trials, bevacizumab was combined with the most active CT regimens in mCRC treatment, including fluoropyrimidines, oxaliplatin, and irinotecan. With a total of 3,007 patients included, 1,864<65 years and 1,142≥65 years old (712 patients were ≥70 years), bevacizumab significantly extended PFS in older and younger patients, with a similar benefit compared to CT alone in all age subgroups (HR 0.59, 0.58, 0.54 for <65, ≥65 and ≥70 age subgroups, respectively). The effect of bevacizumab in OS was not as marked as in PFS in older patients (HR de 0.77, 0.85 and 0.79 for patients <65, ≥65 and ≥70 years old, respectively), while it remained statistically significant and with comparable median OS among all age subgroups. As the authors point out, a higher number of non-cancer-related deaths and more comorbidity in these age groups could partially explain these outcomes. The incidence of the majority of adverse events related with bevacizumab such as bleeding, hypertension, proteinuria, wound-healing complications, fistula, and congestive heart failure were not significantly increased with age.

ATEs and VTEs were more frequent in older people regardless of the treatment arm. However, as far as ATEs is concerned, while its incidence was similar in patients younger than 65 years (2 % in both arms), a higher incidence was reported in elderly patients treated with bevacizumab versus control (6.7 % vs. 5.7 % vs. 2.5 % for patients ≥70 years, ≥65 years and control, respectively). VTEs were 1–2 % higher in patients treated with bevacizumab across all age subgroups, without differences in older and younger people. The incidence of gastrointestinal perforation was <1 % in this pooled analysis, and no definitive conclusions can be drawn with respect to its relative risk on older versus younger patients [6].

Finally, a sub-analysis of the BICC-C study including 117 patients treated with bevacizumab plus irinotecan and fluoropyrimidine combinations in first-line therapy (88 patients ≤70 years old and 29 patients >70 years) showed that OS, PFS, and toxicity data did not differ in both age subgroups, while caution should be taken when interpreting these results due to small sample size. Consistent with the overall results of the study, FOLFIRI plus bevacizumab appeared to be superior to mIFL plus bevacizumab in elderly patients [10].

Analysis of the Observational, Expanded Use Studies

There are two large observational, single-arm trials published to date, the BRITE [11] and BEAT studies [12]. Both tested bevacizumab in combination with different CT regimens in "daily practice" and were carried out in USA and mainly Europe, respectively. A recently published study analyzed the outcomes of elderly patients (≥65 years old) included in BRITE ($n = 896$, 45.9 % of the entire cohort). In contrast to previously mentioned studies, a more heterogeneous elderly population was included, and three cohorts of elderly patients were analyzed separately: 65–74 years old ($n = 533$), 75–79 years old ($n = 202$), and ≥80 years old ($n = 161$). FOLFOX was the most frequently used first-line CT regimen in combination with bevacizumab in all age subgroups, including those ≥80 years old. However, as age was increasing, a higher use of CT regimens not including oxaliplatin or irinotecan was observed. PFS was similar across all age subgroups, but the absolute differences in OS with respect to previously mentioned studies were higher, with medians of 26, 21.1, 20.3, and 16.2 for the subgroups <65, 65–74, 75–79, and ≥80 years old, respectively. In fact, age remained a significant predictor of OS both in univariate and multivariate analysis (after adjusting for baseline confounding factors). However, the study showed that survival beyond progression was similar across age subgroups even when adjusting for confounding factors. Indeed, among others, certain baseline characteristics like performance status (PS), best first-line response, or post-progression CT were unbalanced between older and younger patients (24.1 vs. 12.4 % of the patients ≥80 vs. < 65 years old did not receive therapy beyond progression). These findings suggest that elderly patients with similar baseline characteristics, similar response to first-line CT and with the same treatments received beyond progression obtain comparable benefits to the younger ones. On the other hand, more heterogeneous elderly patients included in this study compared to those included in pivotal trials could also explain the differences in terms of OS obtained in BRITE and RCT trials, respectively. Regarding toxicity reports, the incidence of adverse events related with bevacizumab was similar in all age cohorts, with the exception of a higher rate of ATEs in patients ≥75 years old (4–4.8 vs. 1.4 % for ≥75 vs. <75 years old, respectively). The risk ratio of ATEs for patients 75–79 and ≥80 in comparison with younger patients was 2.85 (IC 95 % 1.25–6.49) and 2.37 (IC 95 % 0.92–6.10), respectively. The risk ratio for the two oldest cohorts after adjusting for possible confounding factors such as PS, hypertension requiring medical treatment, use of anticoagulant therapy, and previous history of ATEs were 2.01 (IC 95 % 0.91–4.44) and 1.67 (IC 95 % 0.64–4.35) [13].

Efficacy and safety data of the elderly patients included in BEAT were presented at ESMO 2009, with 499 and 129 patients 65–74 and ≥75 years old, respectively. Median PFS was similar in all studied cohorts. OS was comparable between <65 and 65–74 years old (23.5 and 22.8 months, respectively) but was lower in patients ≥75 years old (16.6 months). Similarly, a higher incidence of ATEs was reported in patients ≥75 years old [14].

Finally, in a third observational Czech registry, patients treated with bevacizumab in combination with first-line CT regimens ($n = 1,658$, $335 ≥ 65$ years old) found no difference in OS, PFS, or toxicity between patients older and younger than 65 years old [15].

Age-Selected Studies

Studies with Single-Agent CT Plus Bevacizumab

The first study involving almost entirely elderly patients (85 % were ≥65 years) was the previously mentioned AVF2192, published by Kabbinavar and co-workers. Patients considered nonoptimal candidates for first-line irinotecan were randomized to receive 5-FU/LV with or without bevacizumab. Age >65 years was one of the characteristics for inclusion in this trial. Median age was 71.3 months in the bevacizumab group. The addition of bevacizumab to 5-FU/LV was associated with a statistical significant improvement of PFS and RR, and a tendency to an improvement in OS was observed (16.6 months vs. 12.9 months, HR 0.79, 95 % CI 0.56–1.10). It is worth pointing out that two typical toxicities related to bevacizumab such as hypertension and ATEs were apparently increased in this study, in comparison with the bevacizumab arm of the Hurwitz pivotal study. Hypertension was seen in 32 and 22 %, and grade 3 hypertension occurred in 16 and 11 %, respectively. ATEs were described in 10 % of patients with bevacizumab in the Kabbinavar study. Authors suggested that the more advanced age of the population included may have contributed to a higher overall incidence of these toxicities [7].

Three phase II studies have analyzed the safety and efficacy of bevacizumab in combination with capecitabine in front-line therapy of mCRC. The first one included only 16 patients (median age 78 years) and had to be prematurely closed due to low recruitment. Patients were treated with capecitabine at a dose of 1,500 mg/m^2 in a "week on-week off" scheme and bevacizumab at doses of 5 mg/kg every 2 weeks. The median PFS and OS were 9.5 and 21.2 months, respectively, and the most frequently reported adverse events were hypertension (38 % G 2–3) and ATEs (18.7 %). These data should be interpreted with caution, due to the capecitabine schedule and the sample size [16].

The BECA (bevacizumab and capecitabine) study designed by the ONCOPAZ group included a total of 59 patients over 70 years (median age 75 years) treated with capecitabine and bevacizumab in front-line therapy [17]. Significantly, they included patients considered non-suitable for receiving combination therapy with either oxaliplatin or irinotecan, based on Charlson comorbidity scale (a validated method to measure comorbitity based on the presence of illness and its effect on mortality), the level of dependence for basic activities (ADL) and instrumental activities of daily living (IADL), or the basis of a subjective criteria of the investigator. In this regard, it is noteworthy that 13 % of the included patients had ≥ 2 comorbidities according to the Charlson index and 46 % presented a degree of at least moderate dependence (32 % IADL, 14 % ADL). The study did not allow the inclusion of patients on anticoagulants or thrombolytic therapy. The initial dose of capecitabine was determined on the basis of the creatinine clearance (ClCr), in such a way that patients with ClCr≥ 50 ml/min received 1,250 mg/m^2 for 2 weeks followed by 1 week of rest and those with ClCrs between 30 and 50 ml/min received a 950 mg/m^2 dose. Bevacizumab was administered at a dose of 7.5 mg/kg every 3 weeks. The main objective of the study was RR, and the secondary objectives included to determine OS, PFS, and toxicity. With a RR of 34 %, the PFS was 10.8 and 18 months of OS, numerically superior to the data obtained in a similar study conducted by the same group in which patients received capecitabine alone [18]. It is also worth pointing out that 13 patients received post-progression therapies including oxaliplatin or irinotecan. No differences in efficacy in an exploratory sub-analysis made on the basis of the Charlson comorbidity score (0 vs. ≥ 1) were found. The most frequent adverse events (>20 %) were hand-foot syndrome (HFS), diarrhea, asthenia, mucositis, and hypertension, HFS (19 %) and diarrhea (9 %) being the most frequent G 3–4 toxicities. With regard to adverse events related to bevacizumab, the most common was hypertension, mainly G 1 or 2 (19 %). Seven percent of patients developed grade 3 VTEs, but no ATEs were reported. There were five treatment-related deaths, with one gastrointestinal bleeding attributable to bevacizumab [17].

A third phase II study including a total of 41 patients ≥ 70 years (median age 75 years) has recently been published. In contrast to the trial published by Feliu et al., well-defined criteria to determine if patients were or not candidates to receive combination chemotherapy were not assessed. Capecitabine was administered at a dose of 1,000 mg/m^2 for 2 weeks with 1 week off and bevacizumab 7.5 mg/kg every 3 weeks. The primary objective was RR, which reached 65 %. The median PFS was

11.5 months, and the median OS was 21.1 months. Once again, hypertension (49 % G 1–2 and 7 % G 3–4) appeared as the most frequent AE associated with bevacizumab. 12 % experienced G 3 VTEs and 2 % ATEs (1 patient, acute myocardial infarction). The incidence of proteinuria was 5 %. There were two treatment-related deaths, none of them clearly related with bevacizumab [19].

Studies with Polychemotherapy Plus Bevacizumab

To date, data of studies with poly-CT plus bevacizumab in elderly patients are lacking. We have only one trial with preliminary data reported at the American Gastrointestinal Cancer Symposium 2010, which included a total of 48 elderly patients selected for therapy on the basis of the comprehensive geriatric assessment. With a reduced dose of oxaliplatin (100 mg/m^2) every 21 days, capecitabine 1,000 mg/m^2 for 14 days with 1 week off, and bevacizumab 7.5 mg/kg every 3 weeks, the RR was 48 % and no G 4 toxicities or events related with bevacizumab were reported [20].

Conclusions and Recommendations

With the data presented so far (data summarized in Tables 12.1 and 12.2), age alone should not be an exclusion criterion for receiving bevacizumab plus CT in mCRC. Fit elderly patients derive similar benefit in terms of RR, PFS, and OS with the use of bevacizumab plus CT. For those elderly patients not fit enough, less intensive regimen like capecitabine plus bevacizumab is an interesting option, given its convenience of administration, efficacy data, and good safety profile. With regard to toxicity, the most frequent adverse event of bevacizumab in combination with CT in this population is hypertension, but does not have a significantly greater impact in comparison with the younger population. In this regard, bevacizumab should not be initiated in patients with uncontrolled hypertension. Blood pressure should be monitored frequently, especially in those patients with previous history of hypertension. All studies are consistent in establishing that elderly patients have an increased incidence of ATEs with respect to younger ones, and therefore, those with a recent episode of myocardial infarction, stroke, or any other arterial thrombotic event should be excluded from receiving bevacizumab. VTE data are more inconsistent, but in general they seem to have a similar impact compared to younger patients treated with bevacizumab. The rest of bevacizumab-related side effects are also broadly similar in different age subgroups. The incidence of gastrointestinal perforation with bevacizumab is low, and while no definitive conclusions can be drawn, older patients may have a slightly greater incidence compared to the younger ones. Then, those elderly with primary tumor not resected, peritoneal carcinomatosis, previous abdominal/pelvic irradiation, or history or diverticulitis or abdominal abscess should be carefully monitored.

Table 12.1 Efficacy results with bevacizumab plus chemotherapy according to age subgroups

Study	Age (years old)	N	PFS (months) CT+BV	CT+PL	OS (months) CT+BV	CT+PL
RCT nonselected by age						
Kabbinavar et al.	≥65	439	9.2	6.2	19.3	14.3
			HR 0.52 ($p<0.0001$)		HR 0.70 (p 0.006)	
	<65	1,864	9.5	6.7	19.9	16.5
			HR 0.59 ($p<0.0001$)		HR 0.77 ($p<0.0001$)	
Cassidy et al.	≥65	1,142	9.3	6.9	17.9	15
			HR 0.58 ($p<0.0001$)		HR 0.85 (p 0.015)	
	≥70	712	9.2	6.4	17.4	14.1
			HR 0.54 ($p<0.0001$)		HR 0.79 (p 0.005)	
Observational studies			CT+BV		CT+BV	
BRITE	<65	1,057	9.8		26	
	65–74	533	9.6		21.1	
	75–79	202	10		20.3	
	≥80	161	8.6		16.2	
BEAT	<65	1,286	10.8		23.5	
	65–74	499	11.2		22.6	
	≥75	129	10		16.6	
Phase II studies selected by age						
Feliu et al. (Cape+BV)	≥70	51	10.8		18	
Puthillath et al. (Cape+BV)	≥70	16	9.5		21.2	
Vrdoljak et al. (Cape+BV)	≥70	41	11.5		21.2	

PFS progression-free survival, *OS* overall survival, *RCT* randomized controlled trials, *CT* chemotherapy, *BV* bevacizumab, *PL* placebo, *Cape* capecitabine

Table 12.2 Bevacizumab-related adverse events of any grade according to age subgroups

Study	HT	BLD (all)	WHC	ATE	VTE	PRT	GIP
RCT nonselected by age							
Kabbinavar et al. (CT+BV vs. CT+PL)							
≥65 years old	13.8 vs. 1.8[a]	4.8 vs. 3.7[a]	2.4 vs. 0	7.6 vs. 2.8	14.8 vs. 17.5[a]	1 vs. 0[a]	2.9 vs. 0
Cassidy et al. (CT+BV vs. CT+PL)							
<65 years old	15 vs. 4	19 vs. 14	2 vs. 1	2 vs. 2	10 vs. 8	4 vs. 3.7	<1 vs. <1
≥65 years old	15 vs. 4	15 vs. 12	2 vs. 1	5.7 vs. 2.5	12 vs. 10	3.7 vs. 2	1 vs. 0
≥70 years old	14 vs. 4	16 vs. 12	2 vs. 1	6.7 vs. 3.2	13 vs. 10	3.7 vs. 2	1vs. 0
Observational studies							
BRITE (CT+BV)							
<65 years old	1.4	1.8[a]	4.7	1.4	NR	NR	1.9
65–<75 years old	3.4	2[a]	4.1	1.4	NR	NR	0.9
75–<80 years old	1.5	2.4[a]	8.5	4.8	NR	NR	1.4
≥80 years old	3.1	1.3[a]	6.7	4.8	NR	NR	0.7
BEAT (CT+BV)							
<65 years old	27.5[b]	NR	NR	1.1	NR	NR	1.7
65–74 years old	36.1[b]	NR	NR	2	NR	NR	2.2
≥75 years old	29.5[b]	NR	NR	3.9	NR	NR	3.1
Phase II studies selected by age							
Feliu et al.							
≥70 years old	20	7.8	NR	0	7[a]	NR	NR
Puthillath et al.							
≥70 years old	38	NR	NR	18.7	NR	NR	6.2
Vrdoljak et al.							
≥70 years old	56	12[c]	NR	2	12[a]	61	2

HT hypertension, *BLD* bleeding events, *WHC* wound-healing complications, *ATE* arterial thromboembolic events, *VTE* venous thromboembolic events, *PRT* proteinuria, *GIP* gastrointestinal perforation, *RCT* randomized controlled trial, *CT* chemotherapy, *BV* bevacizumab, *PL* placebo, *NR* not reported

[a]Correspond to G 3–4 events

[b]Data given as new or worsening HT

[c]Grade 1–2 nasal bleeding

EGFR Inhibitors: Cetuximab and Panitumumab

Cetuximab (Erbitux®) and panitumumab (Vectibix®) are two monoclonal antibodies against EGFR approved for the treatment of mCRC. Both target the extracellular domain of EGFR, thus blocking ligand-induced phosphorylation of EGFR signaling pathway involved in proliferation, apoptosis, migration, and survival in cancer cells. On the other hand, the KRAS gene encodes a small G protein (RAS) that functions downstream from EFGR-induced cell signaling. KRAS mutations occur in approximately 40 % of colorectal cancers, leading to a synthesis of constitutively activated RAS protein, which is unaffected by the binding of these drugs to the extracellular domain of the receptor [21]. The role of KRAS mutational status as a predictive factor of response and efficacy of these drugs has been definitively established, and their use is nowadays restricted to the wild-type (WT) KRAS population [22, 23]. In recent years, other potential biomarkers of response to EGFR inhibitors involved in this onco-genetic pathway as well as RAS have been investigated. The most important data come from B-RAF mutations. All of them claim that these mutations confer a special poor prognosis in metastatic colorectal cancer but are inconclusive in establishing its predictive role of efficacy or resistance to these EGFR inhibitors in patients with WT KRAS.

Cetuximab

Analysis of Studies Nonselected by Age

Initially, in patients with irinotecan-refractory metastatic colorectal cancer, cetuximab was shown to be active as single agent as well as in combination with the same dose and schedule of irinotecan given at the time of progression [24, 25]. Cetuximab was administered by intravenous infusion at a dose of 400 mg/m^2 followed by 250 mg/m^2 weekly thereafter. Nine percent and 17 % of RR were reported with cetuximab alone or combined with irinotecan, respectively. Toxicities attributable to cetuximab were allergic reactions (3–3.5 % G 3 or 4) and acne-like skin rash (8–9 % G 3) and paronychial lesions, and in the study of combination, other toxicities typically associated with irinotecan were not exacerbated by cetuximab. In both studies, age was not a restrictive criterion for inclusion. In fact, patients up to 83 years old were included. A later randomized phase II trial in irinotecan-refractory mCRC patients, in which cetuximab alone was compared with cetuximab plus irinotecan, demonstrated a significant higher activity in the combination arm (22.9 % vs. 10.8 % RR). Time to disease progression was statistically higher in the combination group, and median OS was better, but did not reach statistical significance (8.6 vs. 6.9 months, $p = 0.48$) [26]. A phase III study in which a total of 572 patients were included (median age 63 years, 41 % ≥65 years) compared cetuximab versus best supportive care (BSC) in fluoropyrimidine, oxaliplatin, and irinotecan-refractory patients. The study showed a statistically significant benefit in OS (6.1 vs. 4.6 months, HR 0.77, p 0.005), PFS (HR 0.68, $p < 0.001$), and RR (8 vs. 0 %, $p < 0.001$). A prespecified subgroup analysis showed that the benefit in OS was independent of age, with similar benefit for elderly patients (5.9 vs. 4.5 months, HR 0.75, CI 95 % 0.56–1.00) to that obtained in the younger group. Skin rash (88.6 %), hypomagnesemia (53.3 %), and infusional reactions (20 %) appeared among the most frequent cetuximab-related adverse events of any grade [27]. Recently a post hoc analysis of this study has been published, with the aim of establishing whether age, comorbidity, or PS are independent predictive and/or prognostic factors for treatment outcome and toxicity. The comorbidity was assessed using the Charlson comorbidity index. As previously mentioned, 41 % of patients included in the study were ≥65 years old, and 25 % of them had comorbidities, with a Charlson index score of 1 in 21 % and ≥2 in 4 % of these patients. In this study, age was not associated with OS in the multivariate analysis, with similar results for patients older and younger than 65 years old (HR 1.21, CI 95 % 0.95–1.55). Surprisingly, comorbidity was an independent factor for better OS in the subgroup of patients treated with cetuximab (comorbidity index ≥1 vs. 0, HR 0.59, CI 95 % 0.37–0.95). These differences did not reach statistical significance in the subgroup of patients treated with BSC. A better PS was significantly associated with better OS both in univariate and multivariate analysis (HR 1.92, CI 95 % 1.34–2.74 for PS 2 vs. 0, respectively). As discussed by the authors, the fact that those with higher comorbidities had better OS resulted in somewhat conflicting conclusions. Among other explanations, they argue that this could be as a result of not correctly distinguishing between PS and comorbidities. Those patients with high comorbidities may have had a better PS than actually attributed, thus biasing the results. Therefore, they conclude that for patients with good PS, restricting cetuximab use in the setting of significant comorbidities is not justified. This study also analyzed data of severe toxicity (≥G 3) according to age and comorbidity. On the one hand, there were no significant differences in toxicity reports between the two age subgroups, with the exception of more dyspnea in patients ≥65 years old (24.5 vs. 11.2 %) and vomiting in <65 years old (7.9 vs. 1.8 %). On the other hand, patients with more comorbidities had less vomiting (0 vs. 7.1 %) but more infection without neutropenia (23.8 vs. 9.8 %) compared to those with lower comorbidities, respectively [28].

The role of cetuximab in second- and first-line treatment has already been established, and in none of these studies, age was a restrictive criterion for inclusion. The EPIC trial included a total of 1,298 first-line oxaliplatin-refractory patients, being randomized to receive irinotecan versus irinotecan plus cetuximab. The median age was 62 years, and patients up to 90 years of age (range 21–90) were included. Combination treatment statistically significantly increased RR and PFS, but OS (primary objective) was similar in both arms. Toxicity was significantly higher for the combination arm for diarrhea neutropenia, and hypomagnesemia. Efficacy and safety data according to age subgroups were not reported [29].

Later on, CRYSTAL [30] and OPUS trials [31] tested the efficacy of cetuximab in combination with FOLFIRI and FOLFOX in first-line mCRC, respectively, and up to 30–40 % of patients ≥65 years old were included. In contrast to previously mentioned studies, efficacy data according to KRAS mutation status was assessed in both of them. Furthermore, an updated analysis of the data according to KRAS mutation status has been published and has consistently demonstrated a significant superiority of cetuximab plus CT in OS (only in CRYSTAL), PFS, and RR in WT KRAS patients [22, 23]. Folprecht et al. analyzed the data of KRAS native patients included in the CRYSTAL and OPUS trials according to age subgroups (younger or older than 70 years). Cetuximab provides similar benefit regardless of the age subgroup. PFS in elderly patients treated with cetuximab plus CT was 8.9 months versus 7.2 months in those treated with CT alone. Similarly, OS was longer for elderly patients treated with cetuximab plus CT (23.3 vs. 15.1 months, respectively). Grade 3–4 toxicity was increased in the elderly in both treatment arms [32].

Finally, in the large phase III COIN trial, cetuximab was combined with oxaliplatin and different fluoropyrimidine combinations (5FU or capecitabine), and efficacy analysis was carried out according to KRAS status. Elderly represented approximately 10 % of patients in each treatment arm. In contrast to previous findings, cetuximab did not prolong either PFS or OS in KRAS native patients [33]. No data on efficacy and safety profile according to age have been reported so far.

Analysis of the Age-Selected Studies

Retrospective Studies

There are two retrospective studies with cetuximab carried out in pretreated elderly patients. In the first one, Bouchahda et al. retrospectively selected a total of 56 patients ≥70 years (median age 76 years, range 70–84) who had progressed on at least two previous CT lines. Eighty-six percent of the patients had received fluoropyrimidines, oxaliplatin, and irinotecan (70 % of the patients with documented resistance to irinotecan), and up to 41 % had previously undergone surgery for metastasis. The majority of patients (96 %) received cetuximab at standard weekly doses in combination with irinotecan at doses of 180 mg/m^2 every 14 days, and not patient was treated with single-agent cetuximab. With a RR of 21.4 %, the median PFS was 4.5 months, and the median OS was 16 months. Any subsequent analysis according to KRAS status was not performed. Treatment was well tolerated, being rash (75, 11 % G 3) and diarrhea (80, 20 % G 3–4) the most frequent toxicities. Six percent of the patients discontinued therapy due to infusional reactions [34].

With a very similar design, Fornaro et al. selected 54 patients ≥70 years old (median age 73 years, range 70–82) treated with irinotecan plus cetuximab in order to assess clinical outcomes according to BRAF and KRAS mutational status. All the included patients had received at least one previous CT line (up to 29 % were >3), and resistance to irinotecan was documented in 100 % of the patients. The treatment comprised cetuximab at weekly dose or 500 mg/m^2 every 2 weeks, together with irinotecan at 180 mg/m^2 every 2 weeks. The RR was 19 %, with a median PFS and OS of 4 and 11.5 months, respectively, in the overall population.

Ninety-six percent of the included patients were assessed for KRAS and BRAF mutational status. As expected, patients with WT KRAS ($n = 29$) obtained a better RR (31 %) and longer PFS (4.21 months) than patients with mutant KRAS tumors (4 % and 3.95 months, respectively), these differences being statistically significant. Although the OS difference did not reach statistical significance (15.82 vs. 10.56, p 0.200), there was a trend to longer survival in the WT KRAS group. None of the seven patients with mutant BRAF (all of which were WT KRAS) responded to treatment, and this mutation was significantly associated with worse PFS with respect to native BRAF patients. The subgroup of patients who most benefited from treatment were those with native KRAS and BRAF. Cetuximab-related toxicity profile was similar to that previously published in other studies with skin rash (87, 15 % G 3–4) and diarrhea (78, 19 % G 3–4) as the most frequent. Thirteen percent of the patients developed neutropenia G 3–4, with 7 % of neutropenic fever. It should be remarked that 39 % of patients required irinotecan-dose adjustment mainly due to G 2 maintained diarrhea and the authors concluded that cetuximab plus irinotecan has an acceptable efficacy and safety profile and compares to previous studies but they suggest considering an initial reduced dose of irinotecan ($130–150$ mg/m^2) in this population [35].

The results of these studies must be interpreted with caution. As the authors point out, these studies have important limitations inherent to their retrospective design and especially with regard to the elderly patients included. Both are mostly composed of heavily pretreated patients who have frequently received previous aggressive treatments, which is reflected in 41 % of surgeries of metastasis carried out in one of the studies and 21.5 % of patients in the second study who received treatment with a triplet (FOLFOXIRI). This is not representative of the majority of elderly patients; thus, many of them have comorbidities and deterioration of the PS that does not allow treatment with so aggressive or long-lasting treatment periods.

Prospective Studies

To date, the evidence of the use of cetuximab in prospective studies exclusively composed of elderly patients is given in trials conducted by the Spanish Cooperative Group for the Treatment of Digestive Tumors (TTD), and all of them were designed before the predictive role of KRAS mutation status was known. The first was a phase II trial whose objective was to determine the activity of single-agent cetuximab as first-line treatment in fit elderly patients. The study was carried out in 2005, when the data for the use of CT in the treatment of elderly patients with mCRC was scarce and with similar efficacy to that expected with single-agent cetuximab. A total of 41 patients were included (median age 76, range 70–88); patients presenting with ≥1 "frailty" criteria were excluded. The primary objective was RR. Several biomarker analyses were retrospectively performed, including EGFR copy number by FISH and the KRAS mutational status. The overall RR was 14.6 %, median PFS was 2.9 months, and a median of 11.1 months for OS was reported. 34 % of the patients did not receive any treatment beyond progression, and a remarkable

percentage of them received only single-agent fluoropyrimidines as second-line therapy. The KRAS mutation status was analyzed in a total of 23 patients whose tumors had sufficient DNA sequencing quality, 18 WT KRAS, and 5 mutant KRAS. Four of the five patients with mutant KRAS had progressed at week 12, while 7 of 18 patients with native KRAS were progression free at that point, although these differences were not significant. The number of EGFR copy numbers by FISH was determined in 36 patients. Eleven patients were FISH+. Forty-five percent of FISH + patients were progression free at 12 weeks including three patients with an objective response. In contrast, only 3 out of 25 FISH-negative patients (12 %) were progression free at 12 weeks ($p=0.04$) With regard to adverse events, skin toxicity presenting as rash and/or folliculitis was the most relevant (70.7 %), 12.2 % of them reaching G 3. The authors conclude that single-agent cetuximab therapy is safe and active in elderly patients with advanced colorectal cancer, but for previously untreated, fit elderly patients should not be an alternative to CT, due to the short PFS obtained [36].

With a similar design and patient profile, another study evaluated the efficacy and safety of the association of capecitabine and cetuximab in a total of 66 elderly patients. The initial dose of capecitabine was 1,250 mg/m^2 for 14 days (950 mg/m^2 if CrCl 30–50 ml/min), but after the first 22 patients included, the dose was reduced to 1,000 mg/m^2 (750 if CrCl 30–50 ml/min) due to severe nail toxicity [37]. KRAS analysis could be determined in the 88 % of the included population. Median PFS for patients whose tumors were KRAS WT was significantly longer than those with KRAS mutant tumors (8.4 months vs. 6.0 months, $p=0.024$). A tendency to longer OS was also observed for patients with KRAS WT tumors (18.8 months vs. 13.5 months, $p=0.107$). Fourteen of 29 patients with KRAS WT tumors responded (48.3 %) compared with 6 out of 29 patients with KRAS mutant tumors (20.7 %) ($p=0.027$) [37].

Panitumumab

At the moment, no studies have been carried out with panitumumab in specific, age-selected patient population. As it happens with cetuximab, age was not an exclusion criteria in the main trials with panitumumab, where >80-year-old patients were included. In the first pivotal study, panitumumab significantly increased the RR and PFS compared to BSC, without significant differences in OS [38]. Later on, a single-arm expanded use trial was conducted, mainly comprising the patients progressing on the BSC arm of the pivotal study, and up to 38 % of the patients were ≥65 years old. Toxicity was very similar to cetuximab, with the skin toxicity as the most prevalent, including erythema, pruritus, acne, and paronychia. There were no infusional reactions reported [39].

Two major phase III trials in first- and second-line therapy, which have combined FOLFOX and FOLFIRI with panitumumab, respectively, have recently been published. In the PRIME trial, FOLFOX plus panitumumab significantly increased RR and PFS in KRAS WT patients, and statistical significance was not reached for OS. Within the subgroup of 656 patients with WT KRAS, 261 (39 %) patients were ≥65 years of age. In this subgroup, there were differences in the magnitude of the effect in PFS for patients <65 (HR 0.70, CI 95 % 0.54–0.89) versus ≥65 years (HR 1.02, CI 95 % 0.75–1.38) (p value for interaction not reported). However, these differences were not reflected in OS (HR 0.80 and 0.81, respectively) [40].

As in first-line therapy, panitumumab significantly increased RR and PFS in combination with FOLFIRI versus single FOLFIRI in the WT KRAS patients, with no differences in OS in the second-line setting. No differences were found between patients <65 versus ≥65 years with native KRAS in PFS (HR 0.69 and 0.87, respectively) nor OS (HR 0.92 and 0.81, respectively) [41]. Although no subgroup analysis with respect to toxicity were done in either of the two studies, tolerance was found to be similar among all age groups and comparable with that reported in those studies of cetuximab plus CT combinations.

Conclusions and Recommendations

Cetuximab and panitumumab seem to have a similar safety profile in the elderly compared to younger patients, either as single agent or in combination with CT. Thus, age alone should not be a condition to exclude the use of these drugs in the mCRC treatment setting. With the limited data available from studies in age-selected patients (Table 12.3), we can conclude that treatment with capecitabine and cetuximab seems to be an interesting first-line combination for patients with WT KRAS tumors, with special attention to the dosage of capecitabine according the ClCr to avoid cumulative cutaneous toxicity. With regard to combined treatments of cetuximab and irinotecan in refractory patients, a lower dose of irinotecan may be used in order to avoid gastrointestinal toxicity. There is no evidence that the major adverse effects attributed purely to these drugs will be increased with age. Skin toxicity occurs in the vast majority of the patients (up to 80 %). In all these studies, the recommended dose adjustment of cetuximab was as follows: When G 3 skin toxicity appeared for the first time, cetuximab was interrupted immediately after toxicity recovered to grade 0 or 1 and then reintroduced at the same dose. After recovering of a second episode of grade 3 skin reaction, cetuximab was reduced to 200 mg/m^2 and after a third episode up to 150 mg/m^2. As far as panitumumab is concerned, the same dose interruption guidelines should be applied with a first reduction of 80 % of the initial dose and a possible second reduction to 60 % of the initial dosage. Skin toxicity should be checked weekly and dose adjustment is mandatory following these recommendations. Diarrhea is one of the side effects potentially increased in elderly population particularly in combination with irinotecan. Patients should be carefully trained for early intervention (oral fluids intake and loperamide) and attend to the emergency unit in the hospital in case of prolonged symptomatology. Finally hypomagnesemia can reach 50 % and should be closely monitored.

Table 12.3 Safety and efficacy data with cetuximab in WT KRAS elderly patients

Study	N	Age	Treatment	PFS		OS		Main toxicities[a] (G3/4, %)
				CT	CT+CTX	CT	CT+CTX	<70 ≥70
Studies nonselected by age								
CRYSTAL and OPUS (KRAS WT population)	845	<70	CT[b] ± CTX	7.7	10	20.2	23.6	Neutropenia: 31 vs. 33
		≥70		7.2	8.9	15.1	23.3	Diarrhea: 13 vs. 23 Skin toxicity 25 vs. 23.1
Age-selected studies								
1. Retrospective studies (pretreated patients)								
Bouchahda et al.[c]	56	≥70	CPT-11+CTX	4.5		16		Diarrhea: 20 Skin rash.: 11 Neutropenia: 1.7
Fornaro et al.	54	≥70	CPT-11+CTX	4.2		15.8		Diarrhea: 19 Skin rash: 15 Neutropenia: 13
2. Prospective studies (first-line therapy)								
Sastre et al.[c]	41	≥70	CTX	2.9		11		Diarrhea: <5 Skin toxicity: 12.2
Rivera/Gravalos et al.	66	≥70	CAPE+CTX	8.6		19		Diarrhea: 9[d] Skin rash: 25[d] Nail toxicity: 7[d] HFS: 7[d]

PFS progression-free survival, *OS* overall survival, *CT* chemotherapy, *CTX* cetuximab, *CAPE* capecitabine, *HFS* hand-foot skin reaction

[a]Independent of KRAS mutation status

[b]FOLFIRI/FOLFOX

[c]Efficacy data not restricted to WT KRAS population

[d]These data correspond to toxicities with reduced dose of capecitabine

References

1. Balducci L, Extermann M. Management of cancer in the older person: a practical approach. Oncologist. 2000;5:224–37.
2. Köhne CH, Folprecht G, Goldberg RM, Mitry E, Rougier P. Chemotherapy in elderly patients with colorectal cancer. Oncologist. 2008;13:390–402.
3. Poon RT, Fan ST, Wong J. Clinical implications of circulating angiogenic factors in cancer patients. J Clin Oncol. 2001;19:1207–25.
4. Hurwitz H, Fehrenbacher L, Novotny W, Cartwright T, Hainsworth J, Heim W, et al. Bevacizumab plus irinotecan, fluorouracil, and leucovorin for metastatic colorectal cancer. N Engl J Med. 2004;350:2335–42.
5. Kabbinavar F, Hurwitz H, Yi J, Sarkar S, Rosen O. Addition of bevacizumab to fluorouracil-based first-line treatment of metastatic colorectal cancer: pooled analysis of cohorts of older patients from two randomized clinical trials. J Clin Oncol. 2008;27:199–205.
6. Cassidy J, Saltz L, Giantonio B, Kabbinavar F, Hurwitz H, Rohr UP. Effect of bevacizumab in older patients with metastatic colorectal cancer: pooled analysis of four randomized studies. J Cancer Res Clin Oncol. 2010;136:737–43.
7. Kabbinavar FF, Schulz J, McCleod M, Patel T, Hamm JT, Hecht JR, et al. Addition of bevacizumab to bolus fluorouracil and leucovorin in first-line metastatic colorectal cancer: results of a randomized phase II trial. J Clin Oncol. 2005;23:3697–705.
8. Saltz LB, Clarke S, Diaz-Rubio E, Scheithauer W, Figer A, Wong R, et al. Bevacizumab in combination with oxaliplatin-based chemotherapy as first-line therapy in metastatic colorectal cancer: a randomized phase III study. J Clin Oncol. 2008;20:2013–9.
9. Giantonio BJ, Catalano PJ, Meropol NJ, O'Dwyer PJ, Mitchell EP, Alberts SR, et al. Bevacizumab in combination with oxaliplatin, fluorouracil and leucovorin (FOLFOX4) for previously treated metastatic colorectal cancer: results from de Eastern Cooperative Oncology Group study E3200. J Clin Oncol. 2007;25:1539–44.
10. Jackson N, Barrueco J, Soufi-Mahjoubi R, Marshall J, Mitchell E, Zhang X, et al. Comparing safety and efficacy of first-line irinotecan/fluoropyrimidine combinations in elderly versus nonelederly patients with metastatic colorectal cancer. Cancer. 2009;115:2617–29.
11. Kozloff M, Yood MU, Berlin J, Flynn PJ, Kabbinavar FF, Purdie DM, et al. Clinical outcomes associated with bevacizumab-containing treatment of metastatic colorectal cancer: the BRiTE observational cohort study. Oncologist. 2009;14:862–70.
12. Van Cutsem E, Rivera F, Berry S, Kretzschmar A, Michael M, Di Bartolomeo M, et al. Safety and efficacy of first-line bevacizumab with FOLFOX, XELOX, FOLFIRI and fluoropyrimidines in metastatic colorectal cancer: the BEAT study. Ann Oncol. 2009;20:1842–7.
13. Kozloff MF, Berlin J, Flyn PJ, Kabbinavar F, Ashby M, Dong W, et al. Clinical outcomes in elderly patients with metastatic colorectal cancer receiving bevacizumab and chemotherapy: results from the BRITE observational cohort study. Oncology. 2010;78:329–39.
14. Van Cutsem E, Rivera F, Kretzchmar A, et al. Safety and efficacy of bevacizumab (BEV) and chemotherapy in elderly patients with metastatic colorectal cancer (mCRC): results from the BEAT observational cohort study. Eur J Cancer. 2009;7(2):349, Abstr 6.088.
15. Kubala E, Bartos J, Petruzelka LB, et al. Safety and effectiveness of bevacizumab (BEV) in combination with chemotherapy (CT) in elderly patients (pts) with metastatic colorectal cancer (mCRC) results from a large Czech observational registry. Gastrointestinal cancer symposium. 2010;Abstr 467.
16. Puthillath A, Mashtare T, Wilding G, Khushalani N, Steinbrenner L, Ross ME, et al. A phase II study of first-line biweekly capecitabine and bevacizumab in elderly patients with metastatic colorectal cancer. Crit Rev Oncol Hematol. 2009;71:242–8.
17. Feliu J, Safont MJ, Salud A, Llosa F, García-Girón C, Bosch V, et al. Capecitabine and bevacizumab as first-line treatment in elderly patients with metastatic colorectal cancer. Br J Cancer. 2010;102:1468–73.

18. Feliu J, Escudero P, Llosa F, Bolanos M, Vicent JM, Yubero A, et al. Capecitabine as first-line treatment for patients older than 70 years with metastatic colorectal cancer: an oncopaz cooperative group study. J Clin Oncol. 2005;23:3104–11.

19. Vrdoljak E, Omrcen T, Boban M, Hrabar A. Phase II study of bevacizumab in combination with capecitabine as first-line treatment in elderly patients with metastatic colorectal cancer. Anticancer Drugs. 2011;22:191–7.

20. Carreca IU, Bellomo F, Burgio SL, Carreca AP, Pernice G, Piazza D, et al. Capecitabine (XEL) and oxaliplatin (OX) in combination with bevacizumab (BEV) in the management of elderly patients with advanced colorectal cancer (ACRC): preliminary outcomes on safety and efficacy. Gastrointestinal cancer symposium. 2010;Abstr 411.

21. García-Foncillas J, Díaz-Rubio E. Progress in metastatic colorectal cancer: growing role of cetuximab to optimize clinical outcome. Clin Transl Oncol. 2010;12:533–42.

22. Van Cutsem E, Köhne C-H, Lang I, et al. Cetuximab plus irinotecan, fluorouracil and leucovorin as first-line treatment for metastatic colorectal cancer: updated analysis of overall survival according to tumor KRAS and BRAF mutation status. J Clin Oncol. 2011;29:2011–9.

23. Bokemeyer C, Bondarenko I, Hartmann JT, et al. Efficacy according to biomarker status of cetuximab plus FOLFOX-4 as first-line treatment for metastatic colorectal cancer: the OPUS study. Ann Oncol. 2011;22:1535–46.

24. Saltz LB, Meropol NJ, Loehrer PJ, et al. Phase II trial of cetuximab in patients with refractory colorectal cancer that expresses the epidermal growth factor receptor. J Clin Oncol. 2004;22:1201–8.

25. Saltz L, Rubin M, Hochster H, et al. Cetuximab (IMC-C335) plus irinotecan (CPT-11) is active in CPT-11-refractory colorectal cancer (CRC) that expresses epidermal growth factor receptor (EGFR). Proc Am Soc Clin Oncol. 2001;20:3a.

26. Cunningham D, Humblet Y, Siena S, et al. Cetuximab monotherapy and cetuximab plus irinotecan in irinotecan-refractory metastatic colorectal cancer. N Engl J Med. 2004;351:337–45.

27. Jonker DJ, O'Callaghan CJ, Karapetis CS, Zalcberg JR, Tu D, Healther-Jane AU, et al. Cetuximab for the treatment of colorectal cancer. N Engl J Med. 2007;357:2040–8.

28. Asmis TR, Powell E, Karapetis CS, Jonker DJ, Tu D, Jeffery M, et al. Comorbidity, age and overall survival in cetuximab-treated patients with advanced colorectal cancer (ACRC)-results from NCIC CTG CO.17: a phase III trial of cetuximab versus best supportive care. Ann Oncol. 2011;22:118–26.

29. Sobrero AF, Maurel J, Fehrenbacher L, Scheithauer W, Abubakr Y, Lutz MP, et al. EPIC: phase III trial of cetuximab plus irinotecan after fluoropyrimidine and oxaliplatin failure in patients with metastatic colorectal cancer. J Clin Oncol. 2008;26:2311–9.

30. Van Cutsem E, Kohne CH, Hitre E, Zaluski J, Chang Chien CR, Makhson A, et al. Cetuximab and chemotherapy as initial treatment for metastatic colorectal cancer. N Engl J Med. 2009;360:1408–17.

31. Bokemeyer C, Bondarenko I, Makhson A, Hartmann JT, Aparicio J, de Braud F, et al. Fluorouracil, leucovorin, and oxaliplatin with and without cetuximab in the first-line treatment of metastatic colorectal cancer. J Clin Oncol. 2009;27:663–71.

32. Folprecht G, Köhne C, Bokemeyer C, Rougier P, Schlichting M, Heeger S, et al. Cetuximab and 1st-line chemotherapy in elderly and younger patients with metastatic colorectal cancer (mCRC): a pooled analysis of the CRYSTAL and OPUS studies. Ann Oncol. 2010;21:Abstr 597P.

33. Maughan TS, Adams RA, Smith CG, Meade AM, Seymour MT, Wilson RH, et al. Addition of cetuximab to oxaliplatin-based first-line combination chemotherapy for treatment of advanced colorectal cancer: results of the randomised phase 3 MRC COIN trial. Lancet. 2011;377:2103–14.

34. Bouchahda M, Macarulla T, Spano JP, Bachet JB, Lledo G, Andre T, et al. Cetuximab efficacy and safety in a retrospective cohort of elderly patients with heavily pretreated metastatic colorectal cancer. Crit Rev Oncol Hematol. 2008;67:255–62.

35. Fornaro L, Baldi GG, Masi G, Allegrini G, Loupakis F, Vasile E, et al. Cetuximab plus irinotecan after irinotecan failure in elderly metastatic colorectal cancer patients: clinical outcome according to KRAS and BRAF mutational status. Crit Rev Oncol Hematol. 2011;78:243–51.

36. Sastre J, Aranda E, Grávalos C, Massutí B, Varella-García M, Rivera F, et al. First-line single-agent cetuximab in elderly patients with metastátic colorectal cancer. A phase II clinical and molecular study of the Spanish group for digestive tumor therapy (TTD). Crit Rev Oncol Hematol. 2011;77:78–84.
37. Sastre J, Grávalos C, Rivera F, et al. First-line cetuximab plus capecitabine in elderly patients with advanced colorectal cancer: clinical outcome and subgroup analysis according to k-ras status from a Spanish TTD Group Study. Oncologist. 2012;17:339–45.
38. Van Cutsem E, Peeters M, Siena S, Humblet Y, Canon JL, Maurel J, et al. Open-label phase III trial of panitumumab plus best supportive care compared to best supportive care alone in patients with chemotherapy-refractory metastatic colorectal cancer. J Clin Oncol. 2007;25:1658–64.
39. Van Cutsem E, Siena S, Humblet Y, Canon JL, Maurel J, Bajetta E, et al. An open label, single-arm study assessing safety and efficacy of panitumumab in patients with metastatic colorectal cancer refractory to standard chemotherapy. Ann Oncol. 2008;19:92–8.
40. Douillard JY, Siena S, Cassidy J, Tabernero J, Burkes R, Barugel M, et al. Randomized, phase III trial of panitumumab with infusional fluorouracil, leucovorin, and oxaliplatin (FOLFOX4) versus FOLFOX4 alone as first-line treatment in patients with previously untreated metastatic colorectal cancer: the PRIME study. J Clin Oncol. 2010;28:4697–705.
41. Peeters M, Price TJ, Cervantes A, Sobrero AF, Ducreux M, Hotko Y, et al. Randomized phase III study of panitumumab with fluorouracil, leucovorin, and irinotecan (FOLFIRI) compared with FOLFIRI alone as second-line treatment in patients with metastatic colorectal cancer. J Clin Oncol. 2010;28:4706–13.

Chapter 13
Palliation and Quality of Life

Bengt Glimelius

Abstract About half of elderly patients with colorectal cancer are left with palliative interventions only due to non-curable disease. Tumor-controlling medical treatment may prolong life and improve quality of life also in elderly patients, but the likelihood of a favorable outcome is less than in younger patients. Multiple subgroup analyses of clinical trials have shown that elderly patients gain as much as younger patients, but selection to clinical trials is extensive and the elderly trial population is not representative of the general population. The transition from a curative to a palliative approach and from when tumor-controlling therapy is meaningful to when it is not are important to consider by the medical staff. The content of the palliative care, for example, not to abandon, be easily available, provide high medical competence, give rapid help, and continue to talk, is as relevant in elderly as in young patients. The aim is to maintain good quality of life as long as possible.

Keywords Chemotherapy • Clinical benefit • Colorectal cancer • Elderly • Palliation • Quality of life

Introduction

In 2012 about 40 % of the patients with a recently diagnosed colorectal cancer (CRC) in the Western world will sooner or later die from their cancer. About half of these are diagnosed with irresectable primary or synchronous metastases, and about half will get a recurrence after a variable time period. The proportion of patients with synchronous metastases is likely higher in older patients, although this is not known with great certainty.

B. Glimelius, M.D., Ph.D.
Department of Radiology, Oncology and Radiation Science,
Uppsala University, Uppsala SE-751 85, Sweden
e-mail: bengt.glimelius@onkologi.uu.se

D. Papamichael, R.A. Audisio (eds.), *Management of Colorectal Cancers in Older People*,   161
DOI 10.1007/978-0-85729-984-0_13, © Springer-Verlag London 2013

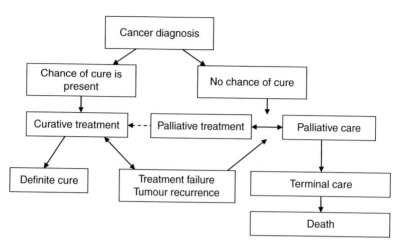

Fig. 13.1 Curative or palliative direction. At diagnosis, treatment direction can be either curative or palliative. Palliative oncology comprises all actions aiming at improving the total life situation in patients who cannot be cured. This period may in colorectal cancer patients vary between a few weeks to many years. Periods of tumor-controlling treatments can alternate with periods where these interventions are not needed or are not meaningful. With improved tumor-controlling therapies, exceptionally good responses may be seen and the palliative intent may turn into a curative intent, although this rarely happens, particularly not in elderly patients. The terminal period usually comprises a limited time period of the few weeks

The delineation between curative and palliative treatment intent is medically rather easy. For most patients the rules of the game are given at the beginning, whether this beginning is at primary diagnosis or in connection with a recurrence (Fig. 13.1). These rules are likely the same independent of age, determined by the stage of the disease and the possibilities of the patient to tolerate the proposed curative treatment(s). The statistical chance for cure decreases with age since the possibilities to deliver the planned curative treatments (chiefly surgery but also neoadjuvant or adjuvant radiation therapy (RT) and chemotherapy (CT)) in a regular way are not always present in an elderly patient. The non-cured proportion thus increases with age. As a consequence, the proportion of patients in need of palliative interventions and care is thus higher among the elderly.

The Cured Fraction and Survival of the Uncured Patients

During the past decades, we have witnessed a substantial increase both in the proportion of patients with CRC that have become long-term survivors, that is, "cured" from the disease, and also in the survival time for those with metastatic disease, that is, of those "uncured." Trials have repeatedly shown that survival in trial patients with metastatic CRC (mCRC) has improved from about half a year to almost 2 years. This difference is, however, an illusion since it is based upon survival of a highly selected group of patients. This selection is particularly evident in elderly patients but also marked in younger patients. When all patients with mCRC were identified in three geographical areas in Sweden, Norway, and Denmark, median survival of trial patients was 21.3 months [1], that is, identical to that of patients included in other trials during the same time period (2003–2006) [2]. Median survival of all 760 patients was, however, only 10.7 months. The proportion of patients that were included in a clinical trial was high (36 %). The proportion of patients receiving chemotherapy was 61 %. These proportions markedly decreased with age, from 41and 86 %, respectively, for below 65 years of age to 0 and 13 % for patients over 80 years, despite attempts not to exclude any patient because of chronological age. Median survival of all patients (trial and non-trial) who received chemotherapy also decreased with age from 18 months below 75 years to 10 months between 75 and 80 years and 8.7 months above 80 years. When survival of those "uncured" or "bound to die from CRC" was modeled in a study based upon the entire Finnish population of CRC, a clear influence of age was also seen [3]. These two population-based results contrast to the finding that elderly patients (>70 years) included in trials benefit from 5-fluorouracil-based chemotherapy as much as younger patients [4]. The latter finding is a reflection of extensive, albeit appropriate, selection for trial inclusion. The elderly patients in general do not yet benefit to the same extent from palliative chemotherapy as younger (<75 years) patients do. With increasing age above about 80 years, the benefit likely decreases substantially.

Cure: At Any Cost

A curative treatment attempt does not always lead to cure. In CRC, as in many other cancers, the statistical chance for cure may vary from let us say 1 % up to almost 100 % between individuals. If the chances are small, it is relevant to discuss whether the attempt is worthy of being named curative but, above all, whether it is motivated in the light of the sacrifice and costs that the treatment can involve. These discussions must be made with the patient, alone or preferably together with significant others, prior to the decision to give up the attempts. A curative attempt may, however, also result in palliation, even if this could possibly have been reached with much less sacrifices. Elderly patients are frequently not prepared to sacrifice as much as younger persons, although there are many exceptions. It is surprising that many very old individuals above, for example, 80–85, are not prepared to give up intensive treatment even if informed about much higher risks of not only morbidity but also mortality from treatments (personal experience).

Palliative Treatment: At Any Price?

Curative and palliative care is essentially quite different. In the curative situation, it may be appropriate to take risks and even expose a patient to severe adverse effects since the gains can be large if cure is achieved. In palliative care, the risks of adverse effects must be limited so that they do not exceed the gains in the form of retained or improved quality of life. These principles are essentially the same whether we are dealing with younger or older patients. The expectations of a continued long life differ, however, for obvious reasons between a young, old, or very old individual.

From Curative to Palliative Care

Even if the intent of treatment is curative, in many instances it sooner or later becomes apparent that the hope of long-lasting disease-free survival must be given up (Fig. 13.1). This change from curative to palliative care is difficult not only for the patient and significant others but may also be so for the staff. When cure is no longer possible, there is a risk that members of the staff feel unsuccessful, although this feeling is likely much less prevalent if the patient is old. Even if these reactions, easy to psychologically understand, may not be particularly common if the patient is old, they must not prevent adequate information to the patient. Since curative and palliative treatments are fundamentally different and since it is the patient who must balance risks and gains of any treatment, it is important not to continue curative treatment motivated by that "it is not appropriate to deprive the patient the hope." This hope mostly means survival. Failure to inform the patient adequately about the transition may easily turn into lack of confidence. The initial aim with the defective openness not to deprive the patient from hope is seldom reached and, even if this may be the case, only for a short time period. At the same time, it is important to stress that the patient irrespective of age not only has the right to know but also has the right not to know.

The Conditions of Hope

The expression "You should never take the hope away from anybody" usually always alludes to the issue of survival. That viewpoint is the perspective of a healthy person. With disease hope will change with conditions. For a cancer patient, the hope to be cured may change to get several years of active life, to be with family and friends for yet a time period, to be at home as much as possible, to that your relatives will master the situation, or to die without pain or other problems. Each of these hopes maybe as important to the patient as the hope to survive once was.

A task of the staff members is to be next to the patient and in a professional way facilitate so that the direction of hope can change with the disease trajectory. It is as important to create good conditions for these changes to occur in elderly patients as in younger patients.

The Content of Palliative Care

Basically, all activities that do not aim at cure or to facilitate cure could be considered as palliative. Thus, palliation is not only end of life care. Survival prolongation is a legitimate aim under the prerequisite that the interventions are performed in consensus with the patient and that the possibilities to treatment success is reasonable in proportion to the activities. Before this weighing of pros and cons is discussed, a few general aspects of the content of activities during the palliative phase will briefly be mentioned. The overriding aim is to try to help the patient to live with as good quality as possible and as long as possible in spite of the cancer.

Do Not Abandon

In many patients there is a fear to be abandoned when curative actions are no longer taken. It is important to actively show that "lots of things can be done" even if cure is no longer possible.

Be Easily Available

In order to actively show that the patient will not be abandoned, the two aspects of being easily available and having continuity are fundamental. One way to show this even for an old cancer patient with comorbidity is that they should have knowledge of who to contact in case of questions or acute problems. It is not appropriate for such a patient to have to contact an emergency unit with no or limited knowledge in the care of the individual cancer patient or cancer patients in general.

Provide High Medical Competence and Give Rapid Help

The relevance of high medical competence among the staff cannot be stressed too much. Rapid help is essential during the palliative phase, particularly if it is in a late phase of the palliative trajectory. All help must be given with very high ambitions. Disturbing physical symptoms can entirely prevent handling of all other problems including the psychiatric and existential ones. It is beyond the scope of this article to discuss the treatment of the many symptoms that may occur. Even if the pharmacokinetics of drugs, like opioids and tranquilizers, may differ between young and old individuals, the treatments and their aims are basically the same. Besides, they are not specific to CRC patients.

Continue to Talk

Besides the medial palliation, it is important to give the patient the possibilities to talk about his or her feelings considering the disease. A short, simple question like "how is it going" together with expressing with your body language that you are prepared to listen and talk as well as consider the patients' emotions can be appropriate. Not all patients are willing or prepared to talk, but the needs are frequently quite high. Somewhat surprising, these talks do not require too much time, sometimes only a few minutes, even if it is an old patient with many concerns and lots to talk about.

Antitumor Treatment as Palliation

During the past two decades, several new drugs have been developed with the aim of prolonging and improving life of mCRC patients. All these drugs, but also surgery and RT, aimed at preventing or delaying the appearance of tumor-related symptoms have adverse, sometimes unpleasant symptoms. It is important to make a balance between these risks from the treatments in relation to those that the disease can create and the likelihood of a meaningful survival prolongation. There is no general recipe of how to make these balances for an individual patient. Most important is that the balances are actively done and that it is the needs and desires of the patient that are satisfied. It is surprising that this weighing is far from always done and seldom properly documented.

The most effective symptom-relieving treatment given to a patient with cancer, including mCRC, during the palliative phase is an active antitumor treatment with no or few adverse effects. There are always reasons for a patient to have problems, even psychiatric, and if the disease that lies behind it can be treated effectively, this should be done. Even if the possibilities to treat mCRC patients for quite some time are large or pretty large, sooner or later the possibilities to control the cancer disappear and only palliative care remains. This "sooner or later" usually comes sooner in elderly patients.

Chances and Risks

In mCRC, multiple trials have documented the proportion of patients who have an objective tumor response according to WHO or RECIST criteria [5]. Besides response, progression-free survival and overall survival are also well documented. The results seen in the trials are based upon the activity of the treatment given but also upon multiple patient-related factors including performance status, many laboratory values, clinical characteristics including types and severity of symptoms, quality-of-life indices, and age. Patients in the trials are always selected to maximize the chances to obtain good treatment results and detect differences in outcome. Several patients in routine care fulfill the inclusion criteria, but many do not, particularly not among the elderly. Actually, among elderly patients, only a minority may be good candidates for chemotherapy as given in the trials. Patients with one or several poor characteristics do worse, sometimes substantially worse than those in the trials, although they may still benefit from treatment [4, 6, 7]. If 40–50 % of the patients respond objectively and another 30–40 % have disease stabilization in the trials, these proportions may easily decrease to 10 and 20 %, respectively, if the patient is 75 years old and has ECOG performance status 2 [8] or is 80 years old with diabetes, slight cardiac morbidity, and performance status 1 [9, 10].

Likelihood of Clinical Benefit

The possibilities of a given treatment to palliate, that is, to prevent or relieve tumor-related symptoms without too much toxicity, are rarely documented. The few studies that have analyzed this most relevant aspect have frequently reported that an objective tumor response is associated with symptom relief if the patient was symptomatic upfront. Disease stabilization, at least if it has a duration exceeding 4 months, is usually also associated with symptom relief [11]. With the type of toxicity that is seen using 5-FU (with calcium folinate, leucovorin) alone, symptom relief was in the majority of patients associated with improvements in quality of life, as measured with a questionnaire [12]. Whether this holds true also for combination chemotherapy, frequently resulting in considerably more acute toxicity, has been analyzed even less. Based upon very limited data, two reviews have stated that quality-of-life outcomes are unrelated to toxicity [13, 14]. When this was analyzed in greater depth in a Nordic randomized trial comparing two irinotecan/5-FU/leucovorin combinations [15], again most patients with a response or disease stabilization lasting for more than 4 months reported improved quality of life. However, a substantial minority (15–25 %) reported deteriorating quality of life [16]. The upper age limit in the trial was 75 years, and therefore, it is not possible to make an evaluation in elderly patients. Since elderly patients, even if in good shape at the start of treatment, more often get severe toxicity and more severe consequences of the toxicity (see below), it can be suspected that the proportion who does not report improved quality of life in spite of antitumor activity from combination chemotherapy is even higher.

The studies including quality-of-life measurements have usually not been analyzed on an individual basis but as group means. For obvious reasons, these mean values represent the average of some patients improved, that is, being palliated; others being rather stable, which may mean palliation if the tumor does not progress; or those who have deteriorated. The proportion actually improved or palliated is thus not properly known. This is even less known in elderly patients even if some studies have indicated that elderly patients included in a trial do as the younger patients do [4, 6, 7]. The possibilities to adequately inform elderly patients of their chances that they benefit from palliative chemotherapy are thus low.

Likelihood of Adverse Effects

The adverse effects of the various treatments are usually known with great accuracy from the trials. The risks of adverse effects in many patients treated in routine care with one or several poor prognostic factors, including increased age, are not properly known, although they are likely higher than reported in the trials. In a pooled analysis of 6,286 mCRC patients, grade III–IV toxicity and 60-day mortality were higher in the 509 ECOG performance status 2 patients [8]. It is also likely that high age per se increases the risk of toxicity, although the extent to which elderly patients metabolize antitumor drugs differently is not properly known [17]. Most trials have failed to control for age-associated changes in organ function. Neither is it known if elderly patients differ in the susceptibility to toxicity from younger patients, although it has been reported that the consequences of toxicity may be higher in the elderly [18]. One study in patients with malignant lymphomas reported that age (>60 years) was of great relevance for hematologic toxicity [19]. The observation phase IV study BRiTE reported that vascular complications to bevacizumab were higher in elderly patients (>65 years) [20]. These patients also had more early deaths. More diarrhea and liver toxicity among elderly were reported in another study of mCRC patients participating in different trials [21]. With this limited information about toxicity to standard chemotherapy against mCRC in elderly patients in general (>75–80 years), it is difficult to inform adequately about the risks if they are not otherwise very healthy.

Taken together, it is reasonable to conclude that most patients above 75–80 years have limited chance to benefit from palliative chemotherapy with a lower probability of response because dose intensity is difficult to maintain. The risk of toxicity is higher than in younger patients, even if dose reductions are done. It is my personal experience that even initially very fit old (>80–85 years) patients are no longer fit after a few months of chemotherapy (5-FU/leucovorin alone or with irinotecan or oxaliplatin), even if their tumors respond well to the treatment. Thus, it may be appropriate to be reserved or very reserved about recommending palliative chemotherapy in this age group. Several readers of this sentence will likely disagree and immediately recall several patients who did well for quite some time. I too have the memory of several such patients during the past decades. At the same time, I and all others have done many more old patients much harm after initiating treatment. We do not see these patients for very long because they have a very short survival, and memory is selective.

Whether the usually small gains in life expectancy from palliative chemotherapy in CRC are worth the potential losses in quality of life from treatment side effects is largely an individual patient choice. Even if adequately informed, many younger and older patients overestimate the chances and underestimate the risks and thus expose themselves to treatments that may do more harm than good.

Importance of Mutual Understanding

It is always of great relevance to achieve mutual understanding prior to initiation of palliative antitumor treatment. This is particularly important in elderly patients where the probability of response and thus clinical benefit is less and the risk of adverse effects higher. In order to reach mutual understanding, it is important to be honest when you inform the patient about the chances of survival prolongation, symptom relief, and the risk of toxicity. The aim should be to give the information in general terms without providing percentages. Many patients still desire active treatment in spite of no chance of benefit and high risks. In these instances it is also important to incorporate significant others in the understanding so that they know the prerequisites. It is actually also relevant to have the hospital staff involved in this information. Otherwise, conflicts may easily appear among the staff. Before the start of treatment, it is also relevant to agree upon when treatment should be finished if it does not give sufficient benefit.

It is also relevant to consider the process that patients go through during a palliative phase. This may alter the patients' opinion either to accept higher risks or the reverse.

The Patient's Right to Refrain from Treatment

Doctors differ considerably in their opinions about palliative chemotherapy, not only in very old but also in younger patients. Looking from aside, it is in many patients easy to see that the chosen treatment is too intensive or in other situations that the activities are too restricted. From aside, it is almost impossible to have a proper opinion about what is behind one or another decision since they are hopefully taken after proper information in heart-to-heart talks. A "wise" decision can only be taken after such talks where the information is directed by the patient. It is my opinion that the desire to initiate antitumor treatment when probabilities of benefit are low is much less if sufficient time has been devoted to the patient, his relatives, and others. It should also be remembered that according to the Swedish (and likely in many other countries) health care law, no patient has the right to demand therapy, only the right to give up a proposed treatment.

Quality of Life

The quality rather than the quantity of the patients' lives is considered to be of the utmost importance. This statement is uncontroversial when it comes to the terminal phase of a patient's life, when life-prolonging treatments are no longer available or not justifiable. It is also uncontroversial if two interventions result in identical survival but differ in subjective toxicity or inconvenience for the patient; the intervention that will result in less effects that negatively may influence a patient's well-being should be selected. The statement is much more controversial if an intervention like palliative chemotherapy may prolong life but at the expense of toxicity that we have learnt negatively influences the well-being of many patients. It is in this situation where the needs for formal measurements of quality of life are the greatest, but also where the methodological obstacles are most prominent. The global questions, considered to be most relevant in the quality-of-life questionnaires to evaluate pros and cons of an intervention, have turned out not to be particularly sensitive to changes between groups and with time [22, 23]. Many mCRC trials exploring different toxic schedules have reported increased symptoms like fatigue and diarrhea, indicating toxicity, but no change in the global measure [24–27]. This lack of change in the global measure to toxic therapy has often been interpreted as if "the treatment was toxic, but it did not deteriorate quality of life of the patients." Coping mechanisms, often designated as a response shift, may well explain this lack of sensitivity [28, 29].

The possibilities to measure quality of life accurately in trials have improved markedly during the past decades [30, 31]. In spite of this, several difficulties remain in the palliative situation when the remaining lifetime is short. Selective attrition is a major obstacle, even if many solutions to this problem have been suggested [22, 23, 32, 33]. In a review of 28 trials in mCRC, most trials considered prolongation of life to be more relevant than influence on quality of life. Actually, quality of life was of overriding importance in only 1 of the 28 evaluated trials [13]. If this is due to methodological problems to measure the highly individual quality of life or is a true reflection of that extension of life is much more important than the well-being of the patients during the remaining life is not known. Even if it is true that many trial patients value the quantity of life more than the quality, we have no good knowledge whether this preference is sensitive to the age of the patient. It is easy to state that quality is more important than quantity of life the older the patient with mCRC treated with palliative chemotherapy is, but it is difficult to find studies that have explored this. Elderly individuals in an apparently healthy population report poorer quality-of-life scores than younger individuals do [34].

Quality of life is highly individual [29]. As a consequence, it has turned out not to be easily measured in palliative, chemotherapy trials. In elderly CRC patients, the presence of several symptoms like pain and fatigue inversely correlates with quality of life [35], and the presence and severity of symptoms are more easily measured than the global or individual aspects. Any medical intervention is also directed toward relieving tumor-related symptoms without causing too many other symptoms. Recording of patient-reported outcomes or quality-of-life measures in elderly CRC patients has however not been frequently done, and this together with only a small number of patients and methodological concerns, particularly patient attrition, seriously limits the abilities to draw conclusions about how treatments affects quality of life in elderly patients [36].

Conclusion

About half of elderly patients with CRC are left with palliative interventions only due to non-curable disease. Tumor-controlling medical treatment may prolong life and improve quality of life also in elderly patients, but the likelihood of a favorable outcome is less than in younger patients. Multiple subgroup analyses of clinical trials have shown that elderly patients gain as much as younger patients, but selection to clinical trials is extensive and the elderly trial population is not representative of the general population. The transition from a curative to a palliative approach and the transition from when tumor-controlling therapy is meaningful to when it is not are important to be adequately considered by the medical staff. The content of the palliative care, for example, not to abandon, be easily available, provide high medical competence, give rapid help, and continue to talk, is of the same importance in elderly as in young patients. The aim is to maintain a good quality of life as long as it is possible.

References

1. Sorbye H, Pfeiffer P, Cavalli-Bjorkman N, Qvortrup C, Holsen MH, Wentzel-Larsen T, et al. Clinical trial enrollment, patient characteristics, and survival differences in prospectively registered metastatic colorectal cancer patients. Cancer. 2009;115:4679–87.
2. Glimelius B, Cavalli Björkman N. Metastatic colorectal cancer: current treatment and future options for improved survival. Scano J Gastroenterol 2012;47:296–314.
3. Lambert PC, Dickman PW, Osterlund P, Andersson T, Sankila R, Glimelius B. Temporal trends in the proportion cured for cancer of the colon and rectum: a population-based study using data from the Finnish Cancer Registry. Int J Cancer. 2007;121:2052–9.
4. Folprecht G, Cunningham D, Ross P, Glimelius B, Di Costanzo F, Wils J, et al. Efficacy of 5-fluorouracil-based chemotherapy in elderly patients with metastatic colorectal cancer: a pooled analysis of clinical trials. Ann Oncol. 2004;15:1330–8.
5. Eisenhauer EA, Therasse P, Bogaerts J, Schwartz LH, Sargent D, Ford R, et al. New response evaluation criteria in solid tumours: revised RECIST guideline (version 1.1). Eur J Cancer. 2009;45:228–47.
6. Köhne C-H, Cunningham D, Di Costanzo F, Glimelius B, Blijham G, Aranda E, et al. Clinical determinants of survival in patients with 5-fluorouracil-based treatment for metastatic colorectal cancer: results of a multivariate analysis of 3825 patients. Ann Oncol. 2002;13:308–17.
7. Goldberg RM, Tabah-Fisch I, Bleiberg H, de Gramont A, Tournigand C, Andre T, et al. Pooled analysis of safety and efficacy of oxaliplatin plus fluorouracil/leucovorin administered bimonthly in elderly patients with colorectal cancer. J Clin Oncol. 2006;24:4085–91.
8. Sargent DJ, Kohne CH, Sanoff HK, Bot BM, Seymour MT, de Gramont A, et al. Pooled safety and efficacy analysis examining the effect of performance status on outcomes in nine first-line treatment trials using individual data from patients with metastatic colorectal cancer. J Clin Oncol. 2009;27:1948–55.
9. Mitry E, Rougier P. Review article: benefits and risks of chemotherapy in elderly patients with metastatic colorectal cancer. Aliment Pharmacol Ther. 2009;29:161–71.
10. Seymour MT, Thompson LC, Wasan HS, Middleton G, Brewster AE, Shepherd SF, et al. Chemotherapy options in elderly and frail patients with metastatic colorectal cancer (MRC FOCUS2): an open-label, randomised factorial trial. Lancet. 2011;377:1749–59.
11. Glimelius B. Biochemical modulation of 5-fluorouracil: a randomized comparison of sequential methotrexate, 5-fluorouracil and leucovorin versus sequential 5-fluorouracil and leucovorin in

patients with advanced symptomatic colorectal cancer. The Nordic Gastrointestinal Tumor Adjuvant Therapy Group. Ann Oncol. 1993;4:235–40.

12. Glimelius B, Hoffman K, Graf W, Påhlman L, Sjödén P-O, Wennberg A. Quality of life during chemotherapy in symptomatic patients with advanced colorectal cancer. Cancer. 1994;73: 556–62.

13. de Kort SJ, Willemse PH, Habraken JM, de Haes HC, Willems DL, Richel DJ. Quality of life versus prolongation of life in patients treated with chemotherapy in advanced colorectal cancer: a review of randomized controlled clinical trials. Eur J Cancer. 2006;42:835–45.

14. Funaioli C, Longobardi C, Martoni AA. The impact of chemotherapy on overall survival and quality of life of patients with metastatic colorectal cancer: a review of phase III trials. J Chemother. 2008;20:14–27.

15. Glimelius B, Sorbye H, Balteskard L, Bystrom P, Pfeiffer P, Tveit KM, et al. A randomized phase III multicenter trial comparing irinotecan in combination with the Nordic bolus 5-FU and folinic acid schedule or the bolus/infused de Gramont schedule (LV5FU2) in patients with metastatic colorectal cancer. Ann Oncol. 2008;19:909–14.

16. Byström P, Johansson B, Bergström I, Berglund Å, Sorbye H, Tveit KM, et al. Health-related quality of life as therapeutic guidance in patients with advanced colorectal cancer receiving palliative combination chemotherapy. Acta Oncol. 2012 (in press).

17. Wedding U, Honecker F, Bokemeyer C, Pientka L, Hoffken K. Tolerance to chemotherapy in elderly patients with cancer. Cancer Control. 2007;14:44–56.

18. Balducci L. Myelosuppression and its consequences in elderly patients with cancer. Oncology (Williston Park). 2003;17:27–32.

19. Ziepert M, Schmits R, Trumper L, Pfreundschuh M, Loeffler M. Prognostic factors for hematotoxicity of chemotherapy in aggressive non-Hodgkin's lymphoma. Ann Oncol. 2008;19:752–62.

20. Kozloff M, Yood MU, Berlin J, Flynn PJ, Kabbinavar FF, Purdie DM, et al. Clinical outcomes associated with bevacizumab-containing treatment of metastatic colorectal cancer: the BRiTE observational cohort study. Oncologist. 2009;14:862–70.

21. Folprecht G, Seymour MT, Saltz L, Douillard JY, Hecker H, Stephens RJ, et al. Irinotecan/fluorouracil combination in first-line therapy of older and younger patients with metastatic colorectal cancer: combined analysis of 2,691 patients in randomized controlled trials. J Clin Oncol. 2008;26:1443–51.

22. Conroy T, Bleiberg H, Glimelius B. Quality of life in patients with advanced colorectal cancer. What has been learnt? Eur J Cancer. 2003;39:287–94.

23. Nordin K, Steel J, Hoffman K, Glimelius B. Alternative methods of interpreting quality of life data in advanced gastrointestinal cancer patients. Br J Cancer. 2001;85:1265–72.

24. Hill M, Norman A, Cunningham D, Findlay M, Watson M, Nicolson V, et al. Impact of protracted venous infusion fluorouracil with or without interferon alpha-2b on tumor response, survival, and quality of life in advanced colorectal cancer. J Clin Oncol. 1995;13:2317–23.

25. de Gramont A, Figer A, Seymour M, Homerin M, Hmissi A, Cassidy J, et al. Leucovorin and fluorouracil with or without oxaliplatin as first-line treatment in advanced colorectal cancer. J Clin Oncol. 2000;18:2938–47.

26. Douillard JY, Cunningham D, Roth AD, Navarro M, James RD, Karasek P, et al. Irinotecan combined with fluorouracil compared with fluorouracil alone as first-line treatment for metastatic colorectal cancer: a multicentre randomised trial. Lancet. 2000;355:1041–7.

27. Bennett L, Zhao Z, Barber B, Zhou X, Peeters M, Zhang J, et al. Health-related quality of life in patients with metastatic colorectal cancer treated with panitumumab in first- or second-line treatment. Br J Cancer. 2011;105:1495–502.

28. Sprangers MAG. Sneeuw KCA Are healthcare providers adequate raters of patients' quality of life – perhaps more than we think? Acta Oncol. 2000;39:5–8.

29. Lindblad AK, Ring L, Glimelius B, Hansson MG. Focus on the individual – quality of life assessments in oncology. Acta Oncol. 2002;41:507–16.

30. Sprangers MA. Disregarding clinical trial-based patient-reported outcomes is unwarranted: five advances to substantiate the scientific stringency of quality-of-life measurement. Acta Oncol. 2010;49:155–63.

31. Efficace F, Bottomley A, Vanvoorden V, Blazeby JM. Methodological issues in assessing health-related quality of life of colorectal cancer patients in randomised controlled trials. Eur J Cancer. 2004;40:187–97.
32. Bernhard J, Cella DF, Coates AS, Fallowfield L, Ganz PA, Moinpour CM, et al. Missing quality of life data in cancer clinical trials: serious problems and challenges. Stat Med. 1998;17:517–32.
33. Moinpour CM, Sawyers Triplett J, McKnight B, Lovato LC, Upchurch C, Leichman CG, et al. Challenges posed by non-random missing quality of life data in an advanced-stage colorectal cancer clinical trial. Psychooncology. 2000;9:340–54.
34. Derogar M, van der Schaaf M, Lagergren P. Reference values for the EORTC QLQ-C30 quality of life questionnaire in a random sample of the Swedish population. Acta Oncol. 2012;51:10–6.
35. Cheng KK, Lee DT. Effects of pain, fatigue, insomnia, and mood disturbance on functional status and quality of life of elderly patients with cancer. Crit Rev Oncol Hematol. 2011;78:127–37.
36. Sanoff HK, Goldberg RM, Pignone MP. A systematic review of the use of quality of life measures in colorectal cancer research with attention to outcomes in elderly patients. Clin Colorectal Cancer. 2007;6:700–9.

Index

D. Papamichael, R.A. Audisio (eds.), *Management of Colorectal Cancers in Older People*,   175
DOI 10.1007/978-0-85729-984-0, © Springer-Verlag London 2013

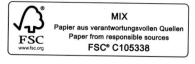

Printed by Books on Demand, Germany